D1471742

How to Incorporate Wellness Coaching into Your Therapeutic Practice

DATE DUE

of related interest

The Insightful Body
Healing with SomaCentric Dialoguing
Julie McKay
ISBN 978 1 84819 030 6

Relating to Clients
The Therapeutic Relationship for Complementary Therapists
Su Fox
ISBN 978 1 84310 615 9

Body Intelligence
Creating a New Environment
2nd edition
Ged Sumner
ISBN 978 1 84819 026 9

Anni's Cancer Companion
An A-Z of Treatments, Therapies and Healing
Anni Matthews
Foreword by Professor Karol Sikora
ISBN 978 1 84819 067 2

Passionate Medicine
Making the Transition from Conventional Medicine to Homeopathy
Edited by Robin Shohet
ISBN 978 1 84310 298 4

Health, the Individual, and Integrated Medicine
Revisiting an Aesthetic of Health Care
David Aldridge
ISBN 978 1 84310 232 8

How to Incorporate Wellness Coaching into Your Therapeutic Practice

A Handbook for Therapists and Counsellors

Laurel Alexander

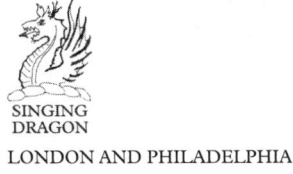

SINGING
DRAGON

LONDON AND PHILADELPHIA

Extract from Medical News Today 2009 on pp.26–27 is reproduced
by permission of Medical News Today.
Extract from International Coach Federation 2010 on pp.68–73 is
reproduced by permission of the International Coach Federation.

First published in 2011
by Singing Dragon
an imprint of Jessica Kingsley Publishers
116 Pentonville Road
London N1 9JB, UK
and
400 Market Street, Suite 400
Philadelphia, PA 19106, USA

www.singingdragon.com

Library of Congress Cataloging in Publication Data
Alexander, Laurel.
How to incorporate wellness coaching into your therapeutic practice : a
handbook for therapists and counsellors / Laurel Alexander.
p. cm.
Includes bibliographical references and index.
ISBN 978-1-84819-063-4 (alk. paper)
1. Health counseling. 2. Health counselors--Vocational guidance. I. Title.
R727.4.A44 2011
362.1'04256--dc22
2011001882

British Library Cataloguing in Publication Data
A CIP catalogue record for this book is available from the British Library

ISBN 978 1 84819 063 4

Printed and bound in Great Britain

Contents

INTRODUCTION 7

Part 1: Setting the Scene for Wellness Coaching 9
Part 1 sets the background to wellness coaching.

Module 1: Emerging Healthcare Trends 11
Growth of the wellness industry 11; The changing face of healthcare 16

Module 2: Integrated Wellness Coaching 29
Defining integrated healthcare 29; The eclectic approach to wellness 30; Definitions of wellness, well-being and health 31; Conventional and complementary healthcare mindsets 32; Areas of life which contribute to wellness 33; The integrated approach of the wellness coach 40; Integrating therapy/treatment and wellness coaching 45; Mindbody integration 46; Integrating limiting client mindsets 54; An integrated wellness coaching example 63

Module 3: Key Issues with Wellness Coaching 66
Differences between coaching, counselling and mentoring 66; Core coaching competencies 68; How people learn 73; Coaching models 76; The importance of client motivation 84; The importance of managing change 89; Wellness coaching networks 94

Part 2: Wellness Coaching Skills Toolkit 99
Part 2 offers a practical toolkit of wellness coaching skills you can begin to integrate into your therapeutic practice.

Module 4: Core Skills Set 101
Wellness Coaching Intro-Pack 101; How to use body language 108; How to use powerful questioning 111; How to use active listening 113; How to develop client rapport 116; How to provide constructive feedback 119; How to facilitate the opening wellness coaching session 121; How to facilitate ongoing wellness sessions 128; How to coach a skill 131; How to end the wellness coaching relationship 132

Module 5: Cognitive Behavioural Coaching   134

Caution! 134; Defining cognitive behavioural coaching 135; The eight-step process to using CBC in wellness coaching 139; Step 1: Setting the scene for CBC 144; Step 2: Problem identification 148; Step 3: Choices and consequences 149; Step 4: Goal selection 152; Step 5: Exploring and challenging faulty thinking 157; Step 6: Decision-making and action planning 175; Step 7: Implementation 177; Step 8: Evaluation 178

Module 6: Additional Skills for Wellness Coaching   180

Biofeedback 180; Stress management 181; Cognitive behavioural coaching (CBC) 181; Relaxation techniques 182; Humanistic psychology 183; Flower remedies 184; Visualization and imagery 184; Nutrition 185; Communication skills 186; Meditation 186; Reiki 187; Pain management 187; Gestalt 188; Emotional intelligence 188; Transactional analysis (TA) 189; Solution-focused brief therapy 189; Rational emotive behaviour therapy (REBT) 189; Environmental wellness 190; Medical qigong 190; Journalling 191; Emotional Freedom Technique (EFT) 191; Positive psychology 191; Neuro-Linguistic Programming (NLP) 192; Multimodal therapy (MMT) 193; Mindfulness-based stress reduction (MBSR) 193

Part 3: Applying Wellness Coaching   195

Part 3 lays out how you can apply an integrated therapeutic coaching approach to specific wellness niches. It assumes therapists have specific discipline-related skills and knowledge and will include these in their wellness coaching practice.

Module 7: Niching Wellness Coaching   197

Choosing a niche market 197; Niche market ideas 202; Creating a diverse business model 213; Your five-step plan to finding your wellness coaching niche 220

Module 8: Applying Wellness Coaching   223

Five ways to deliver wellness coaching 223; Information products 233

Module 9: Marketing Wellness Coaching   239

Consumer buying behaviour 239; What you are selling 243; 62 wellness ideas for wellness coaching 244; Creating a wellness coaching marketing plan 251

LAST WORDS   257

REFERENCES   258

FURTHER READING   264

SUBJECT INDEX   267

AUTHOR INDEX   271

Introduction

This book is intended for complementary therapists and counsellors, or indeed any healthcare professionals who would like to integrate wellness coaching into their existing practice.

I have written this book as a complementary therapist and coach who has a passion for wellness on all levels and who has spent more than 20 years working with adults on issues around physical, psychological and spiritual well-being. Based on my professional experience and tempered by my personal story, I believe now is the time to introduce a wellness coaching book to healthcare professionals and set out a concept that will increasingly become part of our healthcare future.

I am indebted to my clients and students, past and present, who have been instrumental in my development as a wellness professional. While they come to me for healing, knowledge and new skills, one way or another, they have all given me profound opportunities to learn more about how we engage with the process of health and well-being. I see my journey in theirs, and my story in turn gives me the foundation for helping them on theirs.

It is important to say that the wellness journey is not only about prevention or curing; it is often about living with and adapting to progressive disease or preparing for the transition into death. I don't have the ultimate in the definition of *wellness coaching* – it is what you choose to make it. That is what will make you a unique wellness coach. I wish you well in your journey and in facilitating others on theirs.

Setting the Scene for Wellness Coaching

Part 1 sets the background to wellness coaching.

Module 1: Emerging Healthcare Trends

Module 2: Integrated Wellness Coaching

Module 3: Key Issues with Wellness Coaching

Module 1
Emerging Healthcare Trends

By the end of the module, you will have explored:

- The growth of the wellness industry
- The changing face of healthcare

Growth of the wellness industry

We are becoming an ageing, health-conscious mass of humanity. The media bombards us daily with lifestyle concepts for foods, beauty, supplements, diets, plastic surgery, fitness, anti-ageing, self-development and all the rest.

Tongue in cheek, I'm beginning to think we are being conditioned to:

- live to 110 (but look 45)
- have a perfect body (with all bits the right size – whatever 'right' is – and never to drop southwards)
- retain our (perfect) teeth and hair until the end of time
- have no health issues (if we do, we have a network of qualified and compassionate healthcare practitioners to call on whom we can afford or who, better still, don't charge at all)
- eat a balanced and moderate diet (to maintain excellent health and ideal weight while never feeling deprived or bored)
- have wonderfully balanced hormones (zap the PMS and menopause, ladies)
- have sustaining relationships with a range of supportive friends, family and intimates (who are there when we need them but when they're not, we deal with our own issues like the mature adults we are)
- have just the right balance of emotional intelligence

- know what we want, when we want it and how to get it at all times without offending or hurting others

- have a consistently fulfilling work life with a good income (for as long as we are able to stand upright)

- enjoy a regular fitness programme with a happy smile and no aches or pains…

Seriously. Wellness is a growth industry. Why is this? One reason is that we are living longer. People now live on average at least ten years longer than they did in 1948. Illnesses which used to carry us off are no longer killers. For example, tuberculosis was one of the UK's leading causes of death in 1948, killing almost 22,000 people in England and Wales. The rate of death from tuberculosis today is 70 times lower than it was then (Imperial College Healthcare NHS Trust 2011).

Another reason for the increase in wellness is our preoccupation with ageing. Although we live longer, we don't want necessarily to look older, so anti-ageing (or *positive ageing*, as I like to call it) is big business.

A third reason is that many of us deal with chronic or acute health issues on a daily basis, and this prompts us to seek new solutions to make life easier. Fourth is the tendency to move away from pharmaceutical and scientific interventions for health and beauty towards the less invasive and more natural.

Information availability

Business growth is linked to information availability. Over the last 40 years as media technology has improved, we have access to a vast amount of knowledge which has increased our choices related to wellness. Magazines, Internet sites, TV shows, books, radio, CDs, DVDs, CD-ROMs, journals, online forums and chat rooms all offer a window of opportunity to learn more about wellness including self-help techniques, services and products. This has a downside as well as an upside. Becoming better informed is positive; however, being inundated with overwhelming amounts of information, some of it dubious, can be a downside.

The business of health

The business of wellness is multi-faceted. We might separate the arena into products and services, as shown in Table 1.1

Table 1.1 Sectors for wellness products and services

Products

Wellness resources	e.g. informational products, such as an e-Book
Condition-led products	products purchased by or provided to people after they contract a condition; e.g. supplements for irritable bowel syndrome (IBS) or a blood pressure unit
Preventative health-related products	to make buyers feel healthier or look better, to slow the effects of ageing or prevent diseases from developing in the first place
Nutritional products	e.g. supplements, organic foods
Fitness products	e.g. yoga mats, clothing, exercise machines, electronic gizmos
Services	
Wellness coaching	curative or preventative
Lifestyle medical interventions	e.g. botox, cosmetic surgery
Catering	e.g. juice bar or vegan and raw food restaurants
Complementary therapies	e.g. reflexology, homeopathy
Wellness insurance	e.g. personal health insurance and professional insurance for healthcare practitioners
Health and wellness tourism	using travel to experience health and wellness
Commercial fitness clubs	e.g. Virgin Active
Clinically based centres	e.g. those organized by hospitals, GPs and other allied health professionals
Community-based health centres	e.g. Liverpool Community Health (NHS Trust)
Corporate healthcare providers	e.g. Roodlane Medical

There are overlaps between services. For example, some commercial clubs are moving into the clinical arena by offering rehab services. Some community organizations, clinically based fitness providers and commercial clubs deliver corporate wellness programmes. Wellness centres are springing up to provide complementary therapies, personal coaching, fitness and nutrition. Outlets for wellness products exist in all of these outlets, as well as retailers.

There is an inter-industry effect, as one industry affects another. For example, Figure 1.1 shows the effect of the food industry on services and products.

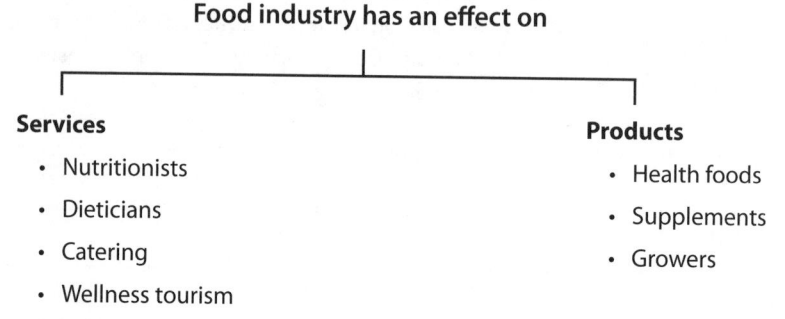

Figure 1.1 The effects of the food industry on services and products

The boom in DIY healthcare

The trend towards do-it-yourself (DIY) healthcare is growing as potential buyers consider how to prevent illness, control health issues, enhance well-being and find ease at life's end. Self-care drives new healthcare behaviours, such as buying information products, wellness tourism (blending well-being and holiday) and purchasing gizmos to use at home or in the office.

Dolly-steps of self-care works with many people, and wellness coaches need to respond to this trend by integrating a variety of healthcare approaches into flexible solutions. Successful lifestyle change requires actionable, individualized solutions and not a one-size-fits-all approach. Buyers don't want to purchase reflexology, exercise or diets. They want to buy solutions for problems. How can I look good? How can I manage my migraine?

Traditional health-club settings are giving way to express workout facilities, yoga studios, medical fitness clinics, speciality yoga (seniors, for example, or bikram) and Pilates centres. The knowledge that exercise improves health also stimulates demand for fitness programmes.

As wellness coaches, we are information brokers, transforming knowledge into individualized wellness coaching programmes and integrating practices from an eclectic choice of disciplines which cover mind, body and spiritual health.

Health sector sales

A couple of financial statistics to whet your wellness coaching appetite:

- The healthcare market in the United Arab Emirates will be worth almost $12 billion by 2015. Around $3 billion will account for wellness products and services sectors. The biggest selling products are anti-ageing treatments (Fenton 2009).

- According to a new healthcare market research report (MarketsandMarkets 2010), the entire home healthcare market covered under the report is estimated to be approximately $159.6 billion. The home healthcare service market is estimated to constitute $143.1 billion in 2009, which is about 90 per cent of the entire market. The home healthcare services market is estimated to reach $207.0 billion by 2014. Home visits and nursing services constitute 72 per cent of the entire market. Most of the growth potential lies in the field of home telemedicine service, which is forecasted to grow at a Compound Annual Growth Rate (CAGR) of 32.3 per cent from 2009 to 2014.

The Golden Boomer boom

A significant portion of the population is now over 55 years of age, and these consumers are a major market segment for the health and wellness industry. One billion children were born between 1949 and 1964, and today these are the 'Golden Boomer' generation. They are called 'Baby Boomers' until they come up to retirement and enter their 'golden years', which begins to happen in 2011.

Concerned with improving their health and maintaining quality lifestyles, the Golden Boomer generation spends on diet fads, healthy foods, supplements and exercise. These consumers are more educated than their predecessors, with a huge amount of wellness-related information available to them. This market segment is interested in improving and maintaining a quality of life and expects vitality long into retirement, when their health and wellness priorities take other forms (e.g. positive ageing, lifelong learning, financial security and retirement concerns).

Mary Furlong, author of *Turning Silver into Gold: How to Profit in the New Boomer Marketplace* (2007), believes that the enormous size of the boomer market translates into vast business opportunities for fitness professionals.

The changing face of healthcare
NHS

Before the state-funded National Health Service was birthed, medical care was a luxury which some could not afford. The NHS was launched after the Second World War in July 1948 and promised to 'care for the British people from cradle to grave' (Beveridge 1942). Between 1948 and 1974, the NHS remained unchanged. Those early years saw the introduction of a charge of one shilling for prescriptions, the revelation of DNA structure and the establishment of a link between smoking and cancer. Since then, all governments have contributed to changing the landscape of health in the UK.

Today, the NHS is still free and offers many services:

- Change4Life advertising campaign (began in 2009) to prevent people from becoming overweight by encouraging them to eat more healthily and exercise more.

- Waiting times of 18 weeks for consultant-led NHS treatment. This means that your treatment should start no later than 18 weeks from the day your GP refers you.

- NHS walk-in services.

- The New Horizons programme, a ten-year strategy to improve adult mental health services in England by 2020, bringing together local and national organizations and individuals to work towards a society that values mental well-being as much as physical health.

- NHS health checks for adults in England between the ages of 40 and 74, reducing the risk of heart disease, stroke, type 2 diabetes and kidney disease.

- Community health coaches who help people to develop healthier behaviour and lifestyles in their own local communities and are employed by a primary care trust.

There is a growing body of evidence to suggest that supporting people to self-manage can improve outcome for service users as well as contributing to capacity across the sector.

A range of longer-term trends also shape the sector. These include the demographic changes in the population, innovations in healthcare provision, the rising incidence and prevalence of people with long-term conditions and the growing expectations of patients themselves. Many commentators believe that these factors now challenge not only the scale of healthcare provision but also the form in which services are delivered. This is unsurprising, since much of the sector and the shape of its workforce is largely based on traditional models of institutions, services and professional groups – many of which predate the creation of the NHS in 1948.

The ageing population and higher life expectancy has led to a growing range of long-term conditions including diabetes, dementia, cancer and arthritis.

These points are applicable to the NHS as well as private healthcare. The key points as I see them applying to wellness coaching are supporting people to self-manage, rising prevalence of people with long-term conditions, an ageing population and personalized care.

The rise of complementary medicine

Complementary medicine has been around for centuries and has gained popularity as a healthcare option. Some definitions of complementary and alternative medicines (CAM) include:

- CAM is a group of diverse medical and healthcare systems, practices, and products that are not currently part of conventional medicine (National Center for Complementary and Alternative Medicine 2010).

- Complementary medicine includes all such practices and ideas which are outside the domain of conventional medicine in several countries and defined by its users as preventing or treating illness, or promoting health and well-being (The Cochrane Collaboration 2010).

- CAM is the non-dominant approach to medicine in a given culture and historical period (Institute of Medicine 2005; a similar definition has been adopted by official government bodies such as the UK Department of Health).

The National Center for Complementary and Alternative Medicine has developed one of the most widely used classification systems for the branches of complementary and alternative medicine. It classifies complementary and alternative therapies into five major groups, some of which have overlap.

- Whole medical systems include alternative medicine built upon a complete system of ideas and practice, such as Ayurveda, chiropractic, homeopathy, naturopathic medicine, osteopathy and traditional Chinese medicine.

- Mindbody interventions are designed to enhance the mind's capacity to affect bodily function and symptoms. These include aromatherapy, art therapy, autosuggestion, flower remedies, Buteyko method, eutony, Feldenkrais method, hatha yoga, hypnotherapy, metamorphic technique, journalling, meditation, music therapy, nia technique, Reiki, self-hypnosis, taijiquan, trager approach, visualization, vivation and yoga.

- Biologically based therapy uses substances found in nature and/or other natural therapy, such as Chinese food therapy, fasting, herbal therapy, macrobiotic lifestyle, diet/food, dietary supplements, exercise, naturopathy, orthomolecular medicine and urine therapy.

- Manipulative and body-based methods are based on manipulation and/or movement of one or more parts of the body; for example, active isolate stretching, acupressure, Alexander technique, anma, bodywork, bowen technique, chiropractic, cranio sacral therapy, Feldenkrais method, manual lymphatic drainage, martial arts, massage therapy, medical acupuncture, metamorphic technique, myofascial release, osteopathy, polarity therapy, reflex point therapy, rolfing, shiatsu, taijiquan, tulayoga, trager approach and tuina.

- Energy therapies are alternative treatments that involve the use of veritable (that which can be measured) and putative (that which have yet to be measured) energy fields such as jin shin jvutsu, magnet therapy, medical qigong, Reiki, shiatsu and therapeutic touch.

Complementary medicine is a mainly private healthcare option. However, many NHS services provide a complementary therapy arm, such as cancer care.

Inside tip

For ten years I was a complementary therapist with a breast cancer care unit in Brighton, Sussex, which is attached to the Royal Sussex County Hospital. The unit would refer patients to me for three one-hour sessions which were free to the patient. I offered reflexology, nutrition, stress management and Reiki. Payment would come from the unit. I worked with primary and secondary cancer patients going through pre- and post-surgery, radiotherapy, chemotherapy and hormone therapy.

Increase in private healthcare

Private healthcare is booming due to convenience and choice, and offers a range of services not routinely offered by the NHS. Complementary and conventional healthcare are offered through the private sector.

Health boutiques, for example, offer one-off treatments such as laser eye correction, dental care, alternative therapies or Botox face-lifts. The idea is to provide this market segment with convenient, on-demand healthcare. Providers are specialized and can provide treatments at a perceived higher standard. In the day-to-day management of lifestyles, people are segmenting their choice of health provider and moving away from mass provision to consumer-led care for the following reasons:

- not wanting to wait for a GP/dental appointment
- not wanting to discuss their issue with a GP
- not wanting a pharmaceutical or invasive solution to their problem
- wanting more time than the allocated slot a GP can offer
- wanting an eclectic approach to their healthcare
- wanting to come at a time that suits them
- not wanting the formality of the NHS.

Private healthcare can be divided into a hierarchy between those who can and cannot afford it. There is a general rule that people from low-income groups may tend towards a higher incidence of illnesses, involving more frequent visits to a GP's surgery or another primary healthcare provider. These patients' accessing private care would involve an unlikely outlay of finances. This embodies a growing need for funded wellness coaching in the community.

With private healthcare in the UK often costing more than most of us can afford, many folks are heading for Europe to get their treatment. Routine dental treatments in France, such as fillings and crown replacements, are cheap procedures when compared to UK rates; The Kontur Clinic in Budapest offers breast enlargements at around £2000 and facelifts at £1700, a fraction of what they would cost in the UK (Izzard 2007).

Private medical insurance increasingly covers a range of both conventional and complementary healthcare options, while many employers offer their staff the option of private healthcare through selected medical care organizations.

Home health services

This change is driven largely by the adoption of telehealth and remote patient monitoring technologies.

Orkney Health and Care and Tunstall Healthcare offer a telehealth service to improve healthcare for patients with long-term conditions. Patients are able to take their vital signs at home under remote guidance (visual and verbal). This results in fewer visits to healthcare centres for routine check-ups. The benefits are numerous: 'Telehealth deployments across the UK have shown that daily health monitoring helps patients to understand their condition, reduce anxiety, and ultimately prevent unnecessary hospital admissions. In addition, increased communication with patients via the phone helps to promote a more preventative approach to the management of long-term conditions' (eHealthNews 2010).

Increasing hospitalization and treatment costs, together with developments in remote monitoring and wireless communications, will create a boom in home-based monitoring, diagnosis and treatment. This trend will also be driven by the rise in the number of people aged 65 and over who are clogging up hospitals. (There has been a 155 per cent increase in the number of Americans being treated for heart failure in the US, not because of an increased disease rate but simply because people are living longer.) The Philips Heart Start Automatic External Defibrillator is a good example of such self-diagnosis or treatment.

Inside tip

During the time I was writing this book, a national charity specializing in health and social care (long-term conditions) phoned me up to discuss the possibility of training key personnel in wellness coaching skills as they gave end-users wellness coaching support by telephone.

Healthcare trends

These are some of the emerging wellness trends of interest to consumers and which should therefore be of interest to you as a healthcare professional.

GIZMO TRENDS

Airload mobile phone

This phone is not only an air filter but also protects its users from viruses and gives off a pleasant scent (Trend Hunter Magazine 2010).

Anti-ageing spa pods

An oxygen bath soothes aches and pains and improves circulation (Trend Hunter Magazine 2009a).

Biofeedback StressWatch

This item tracks your heart rate and body temperature in order for you to monitor your stress responses (Trend Hunter Magazine 2010).

Body Check Ball

The Body Check Ball provides a palm-sized physical including measuring your muscle or body fat percentage and bone density (Trend Hunter Magazine 2010).

Braun's Clever Care Medical Coach
This device reminds you when to take prescribed medicine or supplements, reminds you about medical appointments, synchronizes your medical records and prescriptions from the GP, and provides a database to hold family medical records (Trend Hunter Magazine 2009d).

DuoFertility monitor
The DuoFertility monitor pod can be worn under your arm to learn when you're at your most fertile (Trend Hunter Magazine 2010).

'Memo'
This hi-tech device is designed to be used by those with memory issues. It can send medicine reminders as well as stimulating users with interactive games and providing video conferencing with friends and relatives (Trend Hunter Magazine 2010).

WELLNESS ACTIVITIES
Belonging to spas
Spas are increasingly becoming communities where you spend part of your day and interact socially as well as getting healthy.

Exergaming
Exergaming involves using CDs or video games that track body movement and is used to improve fitness.

Healthy businesses
An increasing number of forward-thinking businesses now include wellness programmes for employees to reduce absenteeism and improve productivity.

Online information
The trend in mobile medical devices is likely to give rise to 24/7 access to medical records (What's Next 2011).

Shoppers spend more on wellness
A new report from The Hartman Group, *Reimagining Health and Wellness* (2010), has found more (mainly US) shoppers have become more inclined to spend money on products aimed at wellness. Since 2005, spending on wellness products shows an upward trend with the average household spending $148.48 per month on wellness-related categories. The report also found consumers seeking more flexible, simple ways of incorporating wellness into everyday life and view indulgence and pleasure as essential to well-being. This most

recent report aligns with previous Hartman Group Wellness Lifestyle Insights reports that pointed to health and wellness no longer being a niche market dominated by a small group of consumers. Consumers across the full spectrum of involvement in wellness can aspire to defining wellness as a quality of life.

Sleeping better
Different products, therapies and programmes are available to fulfil the demand of quality sleeping. Falling asleep faster, sleeping longer and better, waking up refreshed and even getting more beautiful while sleeping are all hot topics. A new term, TATT Syndrome (TATT referring to people who are Tired All The Time), is becoming part of our culture. More people are experiencing sleep difficulties, and to reflect the demands of this sleepless market, new products, therapies and programmes are increasingly becoming available (What's Next 2011).

Time-efficient workouts
Short, intense workouts are designed with time management in mind.

Wellness technology
Technology is entering into wellness initiatives, and there are several new web portals to support fitness, healthy eating and daily activities.

CONDITIONS AND TREATMENTS
Ageing
According to a UN population report, by 2050 the number of adults over 60 years old will surpass that of children under 15 years old for the first time in history. Furthermore, in industrialized countries the number of adults over 60 is anticipated to grow from the 20 per cent observed in 2000 to over 33 per cent by 2050 (United Nations 2009).

According to BCC Research on anti-ageing products and services:

- The global anti-ageing market for the boomer generation was worth $162.2 billion in 2008. This should reach $274.5 billion in 2013, for compound annual growth rate (CAGR) of 11.1%.

- The disease segment generated $66.0 billion in 2008. This is expected to grow at a CAGR of 12.5% to reach $119.2 billion in 2013.

- The appearance segment generated $64.4 billion in 2008. This segment should increase to $105.4 billion in 2013, for a CAGR of 10.4%.

(BCC Research 2009)

Biosimulations
Computers could soon be able to model biological systems and processes, which could then help us to design and test new drugs (What's Next 2011).

Customized treatments
As people become exposed to more wellness-related information and lifestyles become more flexible and complicated, potential buyers are demanding tailor-made healthcare programmes (What's Next 2011).

Depression
Depression is an illness caused by clinical, social (isolation), life event or chronic/progressive conditions which is increasingly being treated in an eclectic way.

Ethics
Many wellness innovations that could drive ethical discussions are coming onto the market; these include brain food for babies, pills that 'do' exercise for us, human limb farms, anti-suicide pills, Viagra for women and age-retarding pills. Cosmetic surgery innovations, including face transplants, voice lifts and bionic eyes, are likely to invoke criticism (What's Next 2011).

External organ helper
An artificial pancreas system using pumps and monitors to improve blood sugar control in diabetes patients has been tested in a medical trial by researchers from Britain's Cambridge University. The system has been shown to keep blood sugar levels within the normal range 60 per cent of the time. Children with type 1 diabetes were given a matchbox-sized monitor and pump fitted with a tube to deliver insulin into the body. The device stabilized blood sugar and reduced the amount of time that blood sugar remained at a dangerous level by half. The eventual goal is a fully automated system that can check patients day and night using wireless data transmission rather than manual control of the pump by a nurse (CBC News 2010).

Medical monitors
Home-based healthcare devices can now provide information about your health to your doctor or healthcare professionals over the telephone.

Memory enhancement
According to US government research, it could one day be possible to download combat experience into the minds of novice air force recruits (What's Next 2011).

Phillips iPill

This vitamin sized capsule includes a microprocessor and a drug reservoir to release medication (Trend Hunter Magazine 2010).

The nurse robot

RIBA stands for 'Robot for Interactive Body Assistance' and was designed by Japan's Institute of Physical and Chemical Research and Tokai Rubber Industries. The nurse robot's foam skin makes interactions comfortable for patients, and is mainly used to assist immobile patients (Trend Hunter Magazine 2009b).

Stick-on stamina

These self-adhesive patches made of water, oxygen, glucose crystals (sugar) and amino acids use the principles of acupuncture to stimulate and improve energy points on the body. There are different patches to help you get rid of pain, increase energy, lose weight and sleep better (Trend Hunter Magazine 2009c).

Health coaching models

Health coaching is the practice of health education and health promotion within a coaching context, to enhance the well-being of individuals and to facilitate the achievement of their health-related goals (Palmer, Tubbs and Whybrow 2003).

We might define *health coaching* as being applicable for existing conditions and *wellness coaching* for curative or preventative purposes. To wet your appetite for integrating wellness coaching into your therapeutic practice, following are some health coaching models from around the globe.

HEALTH COACHING IN GERMAN CONTROL STUDY

A prospective control study was initiated in Germany to observe the effect of whole-patient health coaching on the reduction in hospitalization. The Likelihood of Hospitalization (LOH) prediction model was used to select patients at high risk of hospitalization. Six chronic conditions were identified as criteria for inclusion in the programme. Selected patients were randomized and allocated to a study group or control group. An assessment interview was held on the phone at the outset of the tele-coaching programme to assess patients' current healthcare situation. Patients were subsequently contacted by phone with a view to supporting the client through short-term health improvements (thus preventing stays in hospital), offering such provisions as appointments with specialists, provision of a nurse, training on correct medication intake and regular self-control. Each patient was supervised for six months. The

LOH model was used to select a total of 9176 patients. A control group was comprised of 1080 people. Eighteen months later, the hospitalization rate for the six chronic indications was 25.3 per cent in the study group and 28.3 per cent in the control group. This corresponds to a relative reduction of 10.4 per cent. Conclusion: whole-patient health coaching is a suitable means of preventing hospitalization in co-morbid patients (Stratmann 2009).

HEALTH COACHING WITH BUPA
Bupa offers a telephone-based service facilitated by experienced nurses known as health coaches. The aim is to coach patients in self-management and provide a proactive approach to patient care. According to the organization, 'health coaches are trained to focus on Long Term Condition patients to reduce the likelihood of costly, emergency admission to hospital through lack of self-care' (Bupa undated a).

A COLLABORATIVE CARE MODEL FOR THE NHS
Bupa has a history of working with the NHS to deliver better patient outcomes. Bupa's Collaborative Care Model includes health coaching and allows nurses to target 'risk' patients in order to help them work with their condition in a proactive way. According to Bupa, 'health coaching is fundamental to patients' informed decision-making; clinical support reflects not only individuals' conditions but also their personal priorities, which has the potential to improve patient outcomes' (Bupa undated b).

BUPA PIONEERING HEALTH-COACHING SERVICES IN SPAIN AND FRANCE
Bupa has a central directive of shared decision-making between patients and clinicians. This directive has been shown to 'significantly improve patient outcomes by empowering them to make informed decisions about their healthcare, drive down healthcare costs, and reduce "unwarranted variation" in healthcare interventions' (Bupa undated c). As innovators, Bupa pioneered a pilot in Spain in 2009 offering the country's first health coaching service through the Spanish company Sanitas. In continuation, Bupa expects to offer health coaching services through Spain's national health service as part of an existing partnership including Sanitas' key hospital in Valencia. Bupa has also targeted France, where healthcare practices tend to be driven by medical personnel, and are breaking new ground by offering health coaching to diabetic patients (Bupa undated c).

A PILOT STUDY FOR DIABETES HEALTH COACHING AND MEDICATION ADHERENCE
Health coaching is emerging as a disease management intervention, and has been used in the promotion of medication adherence. A six-month study

evaluated a worksite health coaching model that aimed to improve medication adherence among diabetics. Coaching was delivered via three face-to-face and three telephone sessions, and participants were encouraged to set goals promoting condition management. According to Melko *et al.* (2010), 'the results of this study suggest that health coaching combined with tools to help identify barriers increased medication adherence'.

COACHING TO PATIENT ACTIVATION LEVELS IMPROVES DISEASE MANAGEMENT OUTCOMES (REPRODUCED FROM MEDICAL NEWS TODAY 2009)

People with chronic health conditions who receive coaching tailored to their level of health activation showed significant improvements in clinical outcomes and experienced fewer hospitalizations and visits to the emergency room, compared to those coached using traditional methods, according to a study published in *The American Journal of Managed Care* (an independent peer-reviewed publication dedicated to disseminating clinical information to managed care physicians, clinical decision-makers and other healthcare professionals).

The study, led by Judith Hibbard, PhD, and colleagues at the University of Oregon, compared the behaviours of patients receiving standard telephone disease management (DM) coaching with those who received more tailored coaching based on their 'activation level', as part of a DM programme offered by the health improvement company LifeMasters Supported SelfCare, Inc. Activation levels are determined by the Patient Activation Measure (PAM), a survey tool developed by Hibbard and colleagues to assess an individual's knowledge, skills and confidence in playing a role in one's own health and healthcare.

The quasi-experimental research, which was conducted in a real-life DM setting, included an intervention group and a control group of nurse coaches and their patients in geographically separate call centres, which were selected based on the similarity of their nurse coaches' tenure and years of experience.

The findings show those who received coaching with the PAM experienced a 33 per cent decline in hospital admissions compared to the control group, which remained flat; and a 22 per cent decline in emergency room visits compared with an increase of 20 per cent in the control group. The PAM group also experienced statistically significant improvements in diastolic blood pressure and in LDL cholesterol levels relative to the control group, and increased their adherence to recommended immunization and drug regimens, including the influenza vaccine.

The PAM score intervention group showed fewer hospital stays, which translated into a saving of $145 per person per month for the intervention population. A similar decline was seen in visits to the emergency room among this group, which equates to an $11 per person per month saving.

At the low end of the spectrum, individuals tend to be passive in managing their health and may fail to see the connection between their own behaviours and health outcomes. At the high end, individuals understand that relationship and have become good self-managers across a constellation of behaviours. However, even individuals with high activation levels show opportunities to improve and can benefit from coaching to help stay on course in times of stress or change to their routine.

COACHING PATIENTS ON ACHIEVING CARDIOVASCULAR HEALTH

The Coaching patients On Achieving Cardiovascular Health (COACH) study was designed to determine whether nurses and dieticians who were not involved in medication prescription could coach patients with coronary heart disease to work with their physicians in achieving lower total cholesterol levels and reduction or management of other risk factors. A total of 792 patients from six university teaching hospitals were identified, with 398 being assigned to usual care plus COACH, and 394 assigned to just usual care. COACH participants received regular coaching by telephone and mailing, and it was shown that 'coaching produced substantial improvements in most of the other coronary risk factors and in patient quality of life' (Vale *et al.* 2003).

NHS COMMUNITY HEALTH COACHES

NHS West Essex's community health coaches work with participants over 10–12 weeks to encourage appropriate food and drink intake, increase physical activity and improve sexual health. Links to additional local services are signposted and the service is also accessible through workplace clinics. The service can be accessed by self-referral or by referral from GPs, community nurses, clinics or other health professionals (NHS West Essex 2009).

CPD task sheet

This is your Continuing Professional Development (CPD) task sheet which summarizes key module points and offers you the opportunity to engage with tasks to deepen your learning.

Module summary

- Wellness products can be classified as: wellness resources, condition-led products, preventative health-related products, nutritional products and fitness products.

- Wellness services include: wellness coaching, lifestyle medical interventions, catering, complementary therapies, wellness insurance, health and wellness tourism, commercial fitness clubs, clinically based centres, community-based health centres and corporate healthcare providers.

- There is a boom in DIY healthcare.

- One of the largest markets is the Golden Boomers.

- The face of healthcare is changing with a rise in complementary healthcare as well as an increase in private healthcare and home health services.

- Increasing evidence demonstrates that conventional healthcare systems are using a range of healthcare delivery models.

Your tasks

1. Consider the idea of providing both wellness products and services in your business.

2. Research the DIY healthcare market.

3. Research the Golden Boomer healthcare needs market.

Module 2

Integrated Wellness Coaching

By the end of the module, you will have explored:

- Defining integrated healthcare
- The eclectic approach to wellness
- Definitions of wellness, well-being and health
- Conventional and complementary healthcare mindsets
- Areas of life which contribute to wellness
- The integrated approach of the wellness coach
- Integrating therapy/treatment and wellness coaching
- Mindbody integration
- Integrating limiting client mindsets
- An integrated wellness coaching example

Defining integrated healthcare

We've set the scene for growth in healthcare. Before we move into looking at integrated wellness coaching, let's explore the definition of integrated healthcare.

Many people use conventional medicine for diagnosis before turning to complementary and alternative medicine (CAM), which is used either in place of or in conjunction with conventional medicine. When used in conjunction with conventional medicine, the alternative method of healthcare is called 'integrative medicine' by the National Center for Complementary and Alternative Medicine (NCCAM 2010), because it 'combines treatments from conventional medicine and CAM for which there is some high-quality evidence of safety and effectiveness'.

Ralph Snyderman MD and Andrew Weil MD (2002) state that

integrative medicine is not synonymous with complementary and alternative medicine. It has a far larger meaning and mission in that it calls for restoration of the focus of medicine on health and healing and emphasizes the centrality of the patient-physician relationship.

The British Society of Integrated Medicine (2008) gives the following definition:

> Integrated medicine is an approach to health and healing that provides patients with individually tailored health and wellbeing programmes which are designed to address the barriers to healing and provide the patient with the knowledge, skills and support to take better care of their physical, emotional, psychological and spiritual health. Rather than limiting treatments to a specific speciality, integrated medicine uses the safest and most effective combination of approaches and treatments from the world of conventional and complementary/ alternative medicine. These are selected according to, but not limited to, evidence-based practice, and the expertise, experience and insight of the individuals and team members caring for the patient.

Integrative medicine combines allopathic, complementary, psycho-spiritual and self-help approaches for the prevention and treatment of illness. This includes nutrition, exercise, environmental wellness and our psychological attitude. The underpinning belief is that we abuse our systems because we feel distressed on an 'emotional, social, financial or spiritual' level, therefore our behaviour won't change until we can change our mindset. A foundation stone of integrated medicine is that we can be as involved as we choose in our own healing process, and that the approach of the integrated healthcare practitioner is to encourage and guide our journey (Faculty of Integrated Medicine 2010).

Integrated healthcare could be said to be a self-selected and individually tailored approach to healthcare, combining aspects from conventional and complementary disciplines in order to facilitate the natural healing processes within the client.

The eclectic approach to wellness

Eclecticism is a conceptual approach that does not hold to a single set of assumptions but rather draws upon several ideas and styles to gain insight. This concept forms part of the integrated wellness approach. See Figure 2.1.

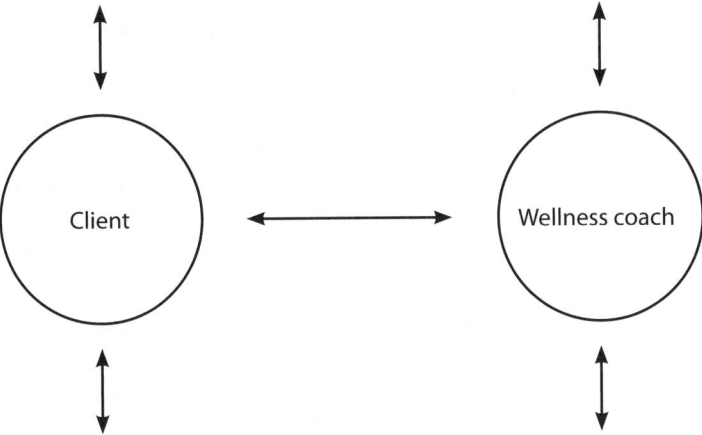

Figure 2.1 The eclectic relationship affecting client and wellness coach and how this influences the coaching relationship

This relationship is a double-edged sword of opportunity for you and your client.

Definitions of wellness, well-being and health

The term *wellness* was first used by the physician Halbert L. Dunn, who published the booklet *High Level Wellness* in 1961. Dr Dunn saw wellness as a lifestyle approach for pursuing elevated states of physical and psychological well-being and described it as a disciplined commitment to personal mastery. He elaborated on a philosophy that was multidimensional, centred on personal responsibility and environmental awareness. Here are some further definitions of health and wellness:

> Health is a state of complete physical, mental and social well being, not merely the absence of disease or infirmity. (World Health Organization 1948)

> We've spent years calling doctors, hospitals, pharmacies and pharmaceutical companies the health industry, when in reality these businesses are truly the sickness industry. The wellness industry is products and services that promote wellness rather than respond to illness – this includes nutritional supplements, super foods and juices, personal trainers and 'alternative care', such as chiropractic. (Pilzer 2007, p.37)

Health is…a resource for everyday life, not the objective of living. Health is a positive concept emphasizing social and personal resources, as well as physical capacities. (World Health Organization 1986)

Health promotion is the science and art of helping people change their lifestyle to move toward a state of optimal health. *Optimal health* is defined as a balance of physical, emotional, social, spiritual and intellectual health. Lifestyle change can be facilitated through a combination of efforts to enhance awareness, change behaviour and create environments that support good health practices. Of the three, supportive environments will probably have the greatest impact in producing lasting change. (O'Donnell 1989, p.5)

Wellness isn't an either/or. A mental or physical, a this or a that. Mending is not the only pathway to wellness. While external sources of treatment may be helpful, they are not exclusive to wellness. It is about the integration of left and right brain, inner and outer truths, life and death, external and internal support systems, mind and body, yin and yang. I would also add that wellness is an organic state and doesn't preclude times of illness. Wellness embraces death as a natural part of life.

Conventional and complementary healthcare mindsets

Conventional healthcare tends to perceive health in a linear way:

Let's identify the problem through tests.

Here are the science-based solutions (pharmaceutical, manipulative or surgical) which you take or we do.

We evaluate the impact of the solution on the problem.

The results are measurable. It is hoped that the problem lessens or goes away. Practitioners of conventional healthcare, looking at the best scenario, might also take into account the person's lifestyle and mindset to create a useful programme. Conventional healthcare has much to offer when used with integrated intent. Most people in the UK have grown up with the 'parental' image of NHS care. We are used to going to the expert for diagnosis and treatment. Our personal inclination then determines how much more proactive we become in our own healthcare.

Complementary medicine (or therapy) refers to methods which can be used alongside or to complement conventional medicine. Some define complementary as alternative, suggesting an either/or belief system. The term complementary and alternative medicine is now often used to include both approaches. The mindset of complementary medicine is holistic. This means the relationship between mind, body and spirit is seen as pivotal to integrated wellness. However, even with complementary healthcare approaches, we can still have the mindset of going to a therapist and giving responsibility to the 'parent' for curing us. Again, our personal inclination determines to how much more proactive we become in our own health.

Challenges

Conventional medicine is relatively easy to access and comparatively easy to do or take. It is tempting for most people to take the quickest route even if it may not be the best route for mind or body.

Not all complementary practices hit the mark, and they might not work quickly. Pharmaceutical practices may lessen or erase the problem, or appear to, and they may work quickly; this is seductive for users. Many complementary approaches, such as whole medical system and biologically based therapies, can provide a 'do to me' approach where clients don't have to get too involved. They take something or change the way they eat, but don't necessarily get more involved. The mindbody interventions require more proactivity and personal investment from the client. Some of the manipulative and body-based therapies, such as the Alexander Technique, require effort from the client.

Wellness coaching requires the client to take responsibility and be proactive. Many people would rather be given something to take or told what to do. We might choose to go one of three different ways here: an entirely conventional medicine route, a totally complementary medicine route, or a mixture of the two – the integrated approach. If we add wellness coaching to the mixture, the process of integration is facilitated by a third non-directive party to whom we can be accountable and yet who can encourage us to be our own healer.

The key challenge for the client is taking responsibility. The key challenge for the wellness coach is inspiring client motivation using non-directive methods while facilitating an integrated process.

Areas of life which contribute to wellness

When we consider wellness, we may start at the point of physical and psychological symptoms. However, our sense of physical and psychological wellness is influenced by other life factors, such as our social interactions, environmental influences, work practices and spiritual beliefs. I'd like you to consider the concept that wellness is an integrated process, as shown in Figure 2.2.

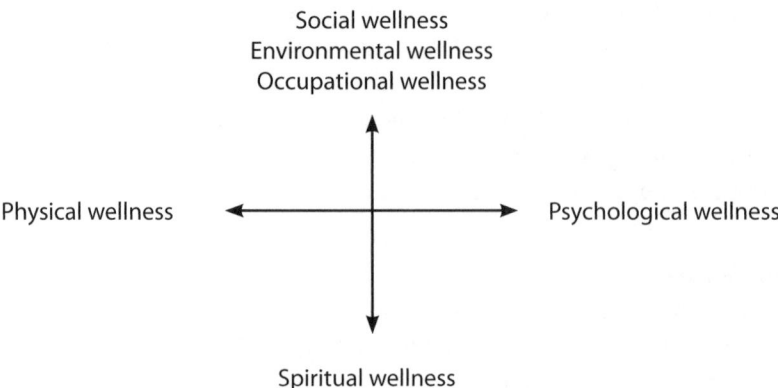

Figure 2.2 *The six areas of wellness are linked*

Spiritual wellness underpins our well-being, but doesn't guarantee our physical or psychological wellness. We might define *spiritual wellness* as our philosophy to ourselves and our relationship with life. Psychological wellness is important in itself and is also key in how we handle physical wellness. Physical wellness (or otherwise) influences our psychological make-up. Occupational, social and environmental wellness impacts us physiologically and psychologically.

Spiritual wellness
While many influences affect wellness, I have put spiritual wellness as the foundation for other areas of wellness because I believe that the wellness of our spiritual nature is crucial to how we live our life, even if we are living with a chronic condition.

We may define spiritual in a religious or philosophical manner. In essence, spiritual wellness can be experienced through a set of guiding beliefs or values that provides a sense of (positive) life direction. The National Wellness Institute gives this definition of spiritual wellness: 'It is better to ponder the meaning of life for ourselves and to be tolerant of the beliefs of others than to close our minds and become intolerant. It is better to live each day in a way that is consistent with our values and beliefs than to do otherwise and feel untrue to ourselves' (Hettler 1976, p.2). When we live in spiritual wellness, we find a sense of harmony between our inner nature and outside forces. We integrate our inner values and beliefs with our external actions.

Think of a ball of light that is constantly moving and evolving. We could say this is our authentic self, our spiritual nature maybe. Imagine a baby blanket covering this ball of light, one of those blankets with a large weave. This blanket metaphorically represents the experience of our human nature, with all its defences and blessings. As we reach for our authentic self (the ball of the light), the light becomes stronger and bigger and pushes the weave apart, letting more and more light shine through. As we peel back the layers of our understanding of our human nature, we allow more and more of our spirituality to shine through on a daily basis. As Socrates said, 'The unexamined life is not worth living'. The spiritual aspect of wellness involves seeking meaning and purpose in our existence. When spiritual wellness is strong, there is strength in times of crisis. We all experience spiritual wellness differently, and each way needs to be honoured.

Inside tips for spiritual wellness

- Spend time alone/meditate regularly.
- An attitude of active searching increases your options and your potential for spiritual centring.
- Trust your intuition – your inner voice will often help you find direction.
- Understand your beliefs, why you have them and why you value them.
- Continue to seek purpose in your life.
- Spirituality is about more than reading; it's about 'doing'.
- Live fully in the present moment.
- Read uplifting books and think about what you read and how to use it in your daily life.
- Acknowledge the fact that you are a spirit with a physical body, not physical body with a spirit.
- Look often into your mind and find out what makes you feel conscious and alive.
- Witness the choices you make in each moment and ask yourself what the consequences of your choice are.
- Take responsibility for your life without blaming anyone, including yourself. See what the situation can teach you and how you can share this teaching with others.
- Practise detachment and recognize uncertainty as an essential aspect of life. Understand that solutions come out of problems and confusion.
- Be playful and find spirituality in music, art, dance, laughter and singing.
- If you notice that certain themes keep coming up in your life, consider the deeper meaning of the pattern. (The Chinese word for catastrophe is the same as their word for opportunity.)

Psychological wellness
COGNITIVE WELLNESS

Just as our bodies need to be exercised and stretched, so does our mind. Mental activities such as learning, problem-solving and creativity are signs of cognitive well-being and are demonstrated through critical thinking. Motivation to learn new things, curiosity plus a desire for self-development are also part of cognitive wellness.

Inside tips for cognitive wellness

- Take a course or workshop.
- Seek out people who challenge you intellectually.
- Read.

EMOTIONAL WELLNESS

To be emotionally well is to have an awareness and acceptance of our feeling nature and how we work and communicate with that. When we are emotionally fit, we feel enthusiastic and positive about ourselves and our life. We understand that the emotional gamut can run from pain to joy and we work resiliently within these boundaries. This work entails taking responsibility and balancing emotional challenge with intelligence and appropriate behaviour in our relationships with others. Emotional wellness involves the meeting of our emotional needs via good self-esteem and appropriate mental healthcare.

Inside tips for emotional wellness

- Tune in to your feelings.
- Spend time with people you trust discussing important personal concerns and being supportive of each other.
- Cultivate an optimistic attitude.
- Learn more about yourself.
- Improve your mood through good nutrition.
- Cultivate an optimistic attitude that includes humour, creativity and faith.
- Engage in regular stress reduction.

Physical (and medical) wellness

Physical wellness is easy to understand because this is the level we are probably the most familiar with. We know that we can experience optimum physical fitness through healthy behaviours such as exercise, good nutrition, abstaining from harmful habits such as drug and alcohol abuse, positive self-care and protecting ourselves from injuries. When we feel as physically good as possible, we enjoy a more positive frame of mind and better self-esteem. In order to experience this level of wellness, we need to take responsibility for ourselves, care for minor illnesses and know when medical intervention is required. Part of our physical wellness programme is medical wellness and involves the appropriate use of conventional and complementary medical systems. According to the Medical Wellness Association (2003), 'Medical wellness is the practice of health and medical care relating to wellness outcomes'. We have a variety of options for disease prevention and treatment; by using a cross-disciplinary medical approach, we can utilize an integrative foundation between conventional and complementary practices to promote the best in wellness.

Inside tips for physical wellness

- Exercise daily or least do some activity for 30 minutes.
- Get adequate rest.
- Listen to your body and learn to recognize early signs of illness.
- If sexually active, practise safe sex.
- Use salt, fat, alcohol and sugar in moderation. Eat breakfast. Eat a variety of healthy foods. Control your meal portions. Eat small but frequent meals throughout the day.
- Get consistent and adequate sleep.
- Stop smoking and protect yourself against second-hand smoke.

Social wellness

Dean Ornish, in his book *Love and Survival* (1999), reviewed scientific literature that showed that adults who related well with their parents, people who have an integrated community of friendships and males who feel loved by their partner all have lower rates of disease and premature death. These findings led Ornish to speculate that social factors may be as important as physical factors in determining overall health.

Social wellness is about a sense of family and friendship as well as local and global community. It involves positive interactions with others and the development of close friendships and intimacy. Social wellness is built on communication skills, caring for others and allowing others to care for you.

Social networks are part of an eclectic approach to wellness, allowing the individual to manage life's problems more easily, thereby easing emotional stress and improving health (Miller 2004).

There are many ways we can support each other. Four clear types of social support have been identified:

- Esteem support: Expressions of confidence or encouragement.

- Emotional support: Physical comfort such as hugs or pats on the back, as well as listening and empathizing.

- Tangible support: Taking an active role for someone else so they can deal with a problem.

- Informational support: Advice-giving, or gathering and sharing information.

Inside tips for social wellness

- Cultivate healthy relationships.
- Get involved.
- Contribute to your community.
- Share your talents and skills.
- Communicate your thoughts and feelings.
- Practise self-disclosure.
- Get to know your needs and pursue a support network which nourishes those needs.

Environmental wellness

Environmental wellness is an awareness of the fluctuating state of the earth and nature and the effects that our daily habits have on the physical environment (home, workplace and the wider environment). It is maintaining a way of life that maximizes harmony and minimizes harm to the environment.

Inside tips for environmental wellness

- Conserve water and other resources.
- Increase your awareness of the limits of the earth's natural resources.
- Conserve energy; for example, switch off unused lights.
- Enjoy, appreciate and spend time outside in natural settings. Renew your relationship with the earth.
- Show care for animals.
- Don't pollute the air, water or earth if you can avoid doing so.
- Minimize chemical use.
- Reduce, reuse, recycle.

Occupational wellness

We will define *occupation* as a paid job or career, or unpaid work such as voluntary or community. Occupational wellness is what you do to give your life meaning and involves choosing work or activities which are consistent with your values, interests and beliefs. Achieving optimal occupational wellness allows you to maintain a positive attitude to use your skills and pursue your goals. When people do what they were meant to do, they deepen their sense of life purpose and so increase their intrinsic wellness.

Inside tips for occupational wellness

- Explore a variety of career or work options.
- Create a vision for your future.
- Choose work that suits your personality, interests and talents.
- Visit a career coach.
- Be open to change and learn new skills.

Integrating lifestyle changes

As we have seen, physical and psychological wellness is influenced by several life areas. These need to be explored, as appropriate, in order to ascertain where changes need to be made. Once these have been identified, you can co-create wellness solutions and support the client in their implementation.

Change management is a part of this process. While clients want to experience wellness in a way that is right for them, making the changes to achieve this outcome can be difficult. Facilitating movement from one state to another requires compassion, realism, flexibility and practicality.

The integrated approach of the wellness coach

Using integrated healthcare as a foundation, we can move into integrated wellness coaching, carrying a similar philosophy.

As a wellness coach, you will work alongside your clients, facilitating their journey towards identified goals and combining several life dimensions of well-being into a quality way of living. You will help your clients:

- make conscious decisions to shape healthy lifestyles

- assume responsibility for the quality of their lives

- adopt a series of key principles in varied life areas which could lead to high levels of well-being and satisfaction

- understand that wellness is the integration of mind, body and spirit

- engage in learning related to their wellness

- understand what motivates them to lead the lifestyles they've chosen

- learn the difference between what they can change and what they cannot, and help them focus their energies wisely

- develop wellness lifestyles which will allow them to revitalize and re-energize themselves, so that they can continue to thrive in the face of ongoing external demands

- learn how to control their thoughts and emotions

- create a sense of connection and meaning in their lives.

Practitioner or client-centred

As a wellness coach, what integrated approaches are you bringing to the coach–client process?

Client-centred therapy (also called person-centred therapy) was developed by Carl Rogers in the 1940s and 1950s and is a non-directive approach to therapy (Rogers 1951). To be directive means the therapist deliberately steers the client in some way, for example closed questions, treatments or making interpretations.

Taking the non-directive approach means that client maintains control over the content and pace of the wellness coaching. The wellness coaching is about whatever the client brings to it. The foundational belief of being client-centred is that clients can find their own answers and therefore move towards wellness. This tendency is facilitated by an accepting and understanding climate which you, the wellness coach, seek to provide, through:

- listening to how things are from the client's point of view

- checking your understanding with the client

- treating the client with respect and regard

- being self-aware and self-accepting (you know yourself and are willing to be known by the client).

Using this approach, the wellness coach facilitates the clients' processes as they discover new things and take proactive steps. Client-centred wellness coaching is a co-creative process of self-discovery and self-empowerment.

As a wellness coach, you participate with clients in their journey by using your knowledge and expertise to understand the client as fully as possible. In reflecting back that understanding, clients hone their awareness of themselves and their own process of wellness. This *non-directive* relationship enables clients to fully experience and express themselves and to authentically *move* within their wellness processes. Your role is one of experienced facilitator or guide, helping clients to clarify and connect with their natural intuition of what feels right, and offering clients a safe space to discover a path that will take them towards where they need to go.

Counselling or coaching

Coaching is problem and solution focused. It deals with the present and future. However, sometimes the barriers to present and future goals have their roots in the past. Occasionally counselling may be necessary to unlock and release the energy so that it might transmute into a coaching opportunity.

If you are a counsellor, you have the opportunity to seamlessly move from a counselling to coaching state. However, you may not feel comfortable doing this. You may need to reflect on whether you want to counsel or coach this client. Boundaries may be an issue for you.

If you are a therapist with little or no experience in counselling, it is important to recognize when you are crossing over from a coaching situation to a counselling situation, and to take appropriate action. The action you might take could include referral or restating the boundaries of the wellness coaching relationship.

People come for counselling because something in their lives is difficult and they need to understand what is happening. In order to understand the present, sometimes the past needs to be explored. The process can be cognitively organic with little emphasis on the practicality of moving on.

A client who seeks coaching comes with a specific problem and may not necessarily be looking for cognitive understanding of the whys and wherefores. They want a solution. Coaching can, however, sometimes touch upon the whys and wherefores so that an emotional discharge can occur and cognitive links made. This link releases the mechanism for moving forward to an outcome. Thus an overlap is formed.

A skilful wellness coach will help clients to acknowledge the past, gain a fresh perspective on it, then form wellness goals which will help them lead a more positive and fulfilled life. The starting point is always the point in the journey where clients are at the time they come to you.

Inside tip

How do you recognize when a client is coaching-ready? A client needs to be emotionally and cognitively ready in order to engage with the wellness coaching process. That isn't to say emotional reactions aren't welcome. But the client does need to be in an emotional space which is relatively easy to self-manage. The client also needs to be able to cognitively balance the books. A client who is emotionally over-reactive or seems unable or unwilling to cognitively engage may not be coaching-ready. This may be the time counselling or going away and metaphorically regrouping may be necessary.

If a client does need counselling, it might be that counselling is needed, lock, stock and barrel. The client may not be ready for wellness coaching at that present moment. These clients can, however, return to you when they are ready. They might require counselling for particular issues and stay with you as their wellness coach for other issues. You could take a counselling qualification or refer the client on (as a total recommendation, or in addition to wellness coaching).

Co-creation

Co-creation is the collaboration between client and wellness coach to create and implement a wellness plan that the client really wants, rather than what the wellness coach wants to sell the client. Your role as a wellness coach is to travel with clients on their journey (not yours), and to facilitate the creative process in ways which are right for them.

It is important that the client does not become dependent on you. It is equally crucial for you not to pick up the mantle of omnipotence and infallibility.

Curative or preventative

As therapists and wellness coaches, is our role curative or preventative – or maybe a mixture of the two?

CURATIVE

When we have something wrong with us, we tend to want instant gratification. We go to the first aid cupboard, chemist, therapist, GP or consultant. We take or do the 'solution'. The discomfort goes away. We mend what is broken. Sorted. Most people will take the easiest path to a wellness solution, which is often a someone or a something. Quick health and fitness gimmicks reap billions annually. Although the curative approach may address the symptoms, it doesn't always sort the root issues of the problem.

Inside tip

I have worked with people on sleeping tablets who want to come off medication. While still on the medication, the clients and I work on creating a toolbox of techniques to help them improve and manage their sleep patterns. When they are ready, with the support of their GP and myself, the clients slowly reduce their medication while implementing techniques from their toolbox. Usually they arrive at a point of no medication and a more controlled sleep pattern. In this instance, the curative is in place while the preventative is being learned.

PREVENTATIVE

A preventative approach to wellness is the step before curative is required, or it may be a step to slow down disease progression. It may be that nothing is broken, or maybe there is a hint of a possible breakdown. Now is the time we can step in to prevent the breakdown from becoming worse. Now is the time your clients can take increased responsibility for their wellness. Clients need to become proactive in order to become informed. When we are informed, we can take action to make changes.

As wellness coaches, preventative delivery comes into play quite extensively as we co-create a wellness plan with clients to suit their needs; these are implemented over a period of time. The preventative approach can also be delivered via workshops and educational settings.

Most people tend not to engage with their health when well. A 'Why mend what isn't broken?' type of mindset. Education plays a crucial role in re-educating mindsets, which in turn can lead to positive behaviours, which influence lifestyle choices. Walking Away From Diabetes pioneered by the NHS is one example. My husband was diagnosed with pre-diabetes. In order to prevent the condition from progressing into diabetes, he attended a half-day course which informed him of the actions he could take to lessen the possible impact of his condition. The course offered information about diabetes and how diet and activity can slow the condition. Since then, it has been his responsibility to change his lifestyle.

People focus on different areas of optimal health as they pass through different stages in their lives because achieving optimal health is a lifelong process. Working with both young people and adults in different life stages can influence our attitudes to wellness and therefore, it is hoped, improve our behaviours in relation to such.

> If all the medicine in the world were thrown into the sea, it would be bad for the fish and good for humanity. (Holmes 1860)

People need to understand the connection between social, environmental, occupational and spiritual areas of their life and how this influences their psychological and physical health. When they make these connections and take responsibility for change, their feelings of wellness (not always the physical condition) often improve.

LIVING WITH A CHRONIC CONDITION

Living with a chronic condition may be partially curative as we work towards alleviating symptoms, but also preventative in relation to slowing down the progression of the condition. In medicine, a chronic condition is a disease that is long lasting. It might be sporadic in its manifestation or gradually worsen over time. Some example of chronic disease include chronic fatigue syndrome, heart disease, arthritis, asthma and diabetes.

Sometimes the word chronic is interchanged with the word progressive. Technically a progressive disease is a physical condition in which the natural course, in most cases, is the worsening of the disease. Some examples of progressive diseases include multiple sclerosis (MS), emphysema, Alzheimer's and macular degeneration.

Chronic disease gives rise to lifestyle changes, such as giving up activities and adapting to physical limitations and special needs. Even day-to-day living may be difficult. Over time, these stresses can rob people of the emotional energy necessary to move forward with their lives. Lack of progress in recovery or worsening symptoms can trigger negative thoughts that heighten feelings of anxiety and sadness. Depression and stress in their turn can exacerbate symptoms connected with the condition. Wellness coaching can play an important role in the management of chronic disease.

PREPARING FOR TRANSITION INTO DEATH

You may be working with an individual who is preparing to die. The client may be in an advanced stage of a disease with an unfavourable prognosis and no known cure, or approaching the end of a natural life span. How we approach death has a lot to do with how we live life, so being the best we can be includes the process of dying as well as living. Dying can be done from a place of wellness. As an experienced wellness coach with insight into this time of sacred transition, you can do much to help clients travel their path.

Integrating therapy/treatment and wellness coaching
Integrating counselling-related activities and wellness coaching

You might be a generalist counsellor, and you may also have specialisms. Areas where you could integrate your counselling experience with coaching might include:

- meeting new people (young, gay, heterosexual, friendship, intimate)
- relationship skills, e.g. assertiveness, anger management, communication skills, conflict management, co-dependency
- positive psychology, e.g. managing perfectionism, change management, improving motivation, emotional intelligence, self-esteem
- life transitions, e.g. menopause, retirement, positive ageing, bereavement
- parenthood
- living with chronic or progressive conditions, e.g. disability
- fertility
- eating disorders
- pregnancy
- addiction
- work, e.g. redundancy, work-related stress, improving work/life balance
- harassment and bullying
- stress, e.g. anxiety, post-traumatic stress disorder (PTSD), depression.

You might specialize in working with men, women or young people and offer one-to-one and group coaching.

Integrating complementary therapies and wellness coaching

Any complementary therapy could be integrated with wellness coaching. You may have experience with specialist conditions which could work with wellness coaching, like pregnancy, positive ageing, fertility, IBS, chronic fatigue, pain management, weight management, high blood pressure or chronic illness.

If you want to blend together a treatment and wellness coaching, you might have time and organizational pressures. This could be done during one longer session or via separate sessions. What does the client need? If it is right to be done in one session, consider whether you start with the treatment or finish with it.

If you don't want to deliver treatment and coaching in the same session but your client has needs for both, the increase in cost to your client might be an issue.

Inside tip

As a Reiki practitioner, I often use Reiki at the start of a wellness coaching session, as this seems to relax and open up the client. If reflexology is required, I tend to use this at the end of the session to bring clients into equilibrium.

It might be that additional therapeutic needs arise from the wellness coaching. For example, you may be a counsellor or homeopath and it transpires through wellness coaching that your client needs to be checked for food intolerances and referred to a nutritionist. This could incur further costs for the client. If you are referring a client, you might want to negotiate preferential rates with your referral partner.

Mindbody integration

Researchers are now increasingly aware that traditional systems of medicine such as Ayurvedic medicine and traditional Chinese medicine incorporate the mindbody link into their practice, whereas Western medicine still tends to view the mind and body as being separate.

Western medicine has moved on and a huge area of research which has been getting increasing attention over recent years is psychoneuroimmunology (PNI). This mouthful of a word can be broken down into psycho, meaning psychology, neuro, meaning neurology/or nervous system, and immunology, meaning immunity. PNI refers to the study of how our psychological states and neurological and hormonal factors affect the functioning of the immune system. Let's have a look at how PNI has developed through a timeline:

- 1884: George Beard, MD, wrote *Practical Treatise on Nervous Exhaustion (Neurasthenia)*, one of the first books to present the idea that the mental state can have a negative impact upon physical health.

- 1909: Richard Cabot, MD, publishes his *Social Service and the Art of Healing* and wrote:

  I found myself constantly baffled and discouraged when it came to treatment. Treatment in more than half of the cases... involved an understanding of the patient's economic situation and economic means, but still more of his mentality, his character, his previous mental and industrial history, all that brought him to his present condition in which sickness, fear, worry, and poverty were found inextricably mingled.

- 1920s: Dr Cannon coined the phrase 'fight or flight response' (1915) when he discovered the relationship between the stress of perceived danger and neuroendocrine responses in animals. Cannon also coined the term *homeostasis*, from the Greek word *homoios* meaning similar, and *stasis* meaning position, and presented it in his book *The Wisdom of the Body* (1932). Human homeostasis refers to the body's ability to physiologically regulate its inner environment to ensure its stability in response to fluctuations in the outside environment.

- 1934: Joseph Pilates publishes *Your Health* (1998/1934). In 1945 he wrote *Return to Life Through Contrology* with William John Miller (1998/1945) about the stresses of modern life. Pilates wrote on issues such as the mindbody connection, wellness, the benefits of mindbody exercise, and functional exercise.

- 1936: Hans Selye coined the phrase 'General Adaptation Syndrome' where stressors such as hot and cold produce a generalized response in biological organisms as they respond with automatic somatic reactions.

- 1938: Dr Jacobson, in *Progressive Relaxation*, developed a relaxation technique that claimed anxiety is caused by skeletal muscle contractions.

- 1940s: Harold Wolff moved from Cannon's fight-or-flight self-defence disease model to a more generalized notion of stress and disease where people respond to stressful situations or events (Wolff 1953).

- 1950s: Hans Selye became the best-known proponent of the role played by stress in psychosomatic theory (Selye 1956, 1973, 1974).

- 1961: Halbert Dunn published *High Level Wellness*. Wellness comes to mean a new concept in which health is more than absence of disease. *Wellness* now refers to a healthy balance of the mind, body and spirit that results in an overall feeling of well-being.

- 1964: Psychiatrist George Solomon noticed that people with rheumatoid arthritis got worse when they were depressed. He began to investigate the impact emotions had on inflammation and the immune system in general. He coined the term *psychoimmunology* and published a paper, 'Emotions, immunity, and disease: A speculative theoretical integration' (Solomon and Moos 1964).

- 1969: Neil Miller, a pioneer in biofeedback research, showed that it was possible to apply the principles of operatant behaviour shaping towards altering internal bodily functions like heart rate. Miller's 'visceral learning' would later come to be known as *biofeedback*. Miller established that we can learn to control our autonomic nervous system.

- 1970s: The term 'behavioural medicine' was coined by Birk (1973) when discussing the virtues of biofeedback.

- 1974: Herbert Benson coined the phrase 'relaxation response'. Benson viewed the relaxation response as being opposite to the fight-or-flight response. Both of these responses involved physiological changes in the brain's hypothalamus. The fight-or-flight response provokes feelings of anxiety and increased levels of blood-lactate. The relaxation response was presented as a method more practical than biofeedback that effectively counters inappropriate elicitation of the fight-or-flight response (Benson 1975; Benson, Beary and Carol 1974).

- 1975: Psychologist Robert Ader and immunologist Nicholas Cohen at the University of Rochester Medical Centre in Rochester, New York, advanced PNI with their demonstration of classic conditioning of immune function, and coined the term *psychoneuroimmunology*. Ader showed that mental and emotional cues could affect the immune system. In the 1970s, studies by Ader and other researchers opened up new understandings of how experiences such as stress can affect a person's immune system. In particular, this was borne out in a study conducted by Ader and his colleagues which showed that it is possible to classically condition the immune system. Following extensive research, he suggested that depression can be interpreted by the body to produce lethargy and other corresponding ailments. Conversely, if the body is diagnosed with a serious disease like cancer, a negative mental state may ensue.

- 1977: George Engel, MD, first proposed the biopsychosocial model of health, wellness and illness which sees health, illness and healing as resulting from the interacting effects of events of different types, including biological, psychological and social factors. All of these are seen as systems that affect one another and interact with one another to affect individual health.

- 1981: Leading researcher and neurobiologist Dr David Felten (Indiana University of Medicine) made some of the first links on neuroimmune interactions. Research uncovered a network of nerves leading to the cells of the immune system and blood vessels. Further research identified nerves in the spleen and thymus which terminated close to clusters of lymphocytes, macrophages and mast cells (related to immune function) (Rochester Review 1997).

- 1981: Ader, Cohen and Felten edited the book *Psychoneuroimmunology* which laid out the underlying premise that the brain and immune system represent a single integrated system of defence. (An updated fourth edition was released in 2006.)

- 1985: Research by neuropharmacologist Candace Pert (Pert *et al.* 1985) showed that natural chemicals called neuropeptide-specific receptors are present on the cell walls of both the brain and the immune system. These substances not only act directly on the immune system but also on our emotions and suggest mechanisms through which emotions and immunology are interdependent. As these complex messengers travel throughout the body, they provide vital information and sometimes almost instant physical feedback. When you come up against something frightening, you might have a physical reaction like shaking. This shows how fast information can be transmitted from thought to physiology. This emotional creation requires input from the brain, specifically the limbic system and the hypothalamus. The discovery by Pert, that neuropeptides and neurotransmitters are also on cell walls of the immune system, shows a close association with emotions and suggests that emotions and health are interdependent (Ruff *et al.* 1985). This demonstration that the immune and endocrine systems are modulated not only by the brain but by the central nervous system itself has had an impact on how we understand the mindbody connection.

There is sufficient data to conclude that immune system function can be influenced by psychosocial stressors which can lead to physiological changes. There are possible pathways from psychological stress to physical distress. Faulty thinking can lead to emotional turmoil, which may produce inappropriate behaviour, for example over-eating or workaholism. Evidence seems to suggest that a loss of psychological control can lead to a reduction of normal homeostasis; when this happens, our immune system is weakened making it easier for symptoms to manifest.

How a person deals with emotions may affect how long they survive with a chronic illness. The goal of mindbody techniques is to get the body and mind to relax and to reduce the levels of stress hormones in the body, so the immune system is better able to fight off illness. Mindbody techniques can be helpful for many conditions because they encourage relaxation, improve coping skills, reduce tension and pain, and lessen the need for medication. For example, mindbody techniques like meditation and imagery are used along with medication to treat pain. Symptoms of anxiety and depression also respond well to mindbody techniques. Mindbody techniques may help treat many different conditions, including high blood pressure, asthma, heart disease, tinnitus, pain and nausea related to chemotherapy, insomnia, anxiety, digestive problems and fibromyalgia.

Allopathic interventions have made fantastic advances. However, in order to move into the 21st century, healthcare now needs to make allowances for emotional well-being in an integrated healthcare approach.

The stress factor

As part of our exploration on the mindbody link, let's focus on stress.

Stress isn't caused by any one event. It more describes our response to an event. The same event can happen to two people, and one may respond with a high level of stress symptoms while the other deals with the situation without any stress symptoms. Our perception of the event and our coping strategies determine how 'stressed' we become. Positive stress adds the edge of anticipation to life. We don't want to eliminate stress but learn how to manage it. See Table 2.1 for an outline of the different signs of stress.

ACUTE AND CHRONIC STRESS

Acute stress results from an acute situation and is the reaction to an immediate threat, known as the fight-or-flight response. The threat can be any situation that is experienced as a danger. Symptoms include tension headaches, feelings of agitation and pressure and gastrointestinal disturbances. Under most circumstances, once the acute threat has passed, the response becomes inactivated and levels of stress hormones return to normal, a condition called the *relaxation response*. Sometimes the event has a positive outcome; the stress passes and we move on. But if the stressful event doesn't pass or is immediately followed by another stressful event, the acute stress can become what's known as *episodic*. Symptoms might include migraines, hypertension, stroke, heart

Table 2.1 Signs of stress	
Physical signs of stress	increased heart rate, sweaty palms, headache, muscular tightness, diarrhoea/constipation, nausea, sleep disturbances, fatigue, shallow breathing, dryness of mouth, recurrent viral illnesses/infections, stomach ulcers, high blood pressure, chest pain and loss of/increased appetite
Emotional signs of stress	irritability, angry outbursts, depression, feelings of unreality, narrowed focus, reduced self-esteem, decreased perception of positive, and anxiety
Cognitive signs of stress	forgetfulness, reduced creativity, lack of concentration, disorganization of thought, diminished sense of meaning in life and negative self-talk
Behavioural signs of stress	carelessness, increased smoking/alcohol/drug use, withdrawal, listlessness, nervous laughter, accident proneness, nail biting, aggressive behaviour, e.g. road rage and grinding teeth

attack, anxiety, depression or serious gastrointestinal distress, which can take longer to recover from. Workaholics and those with type-A personalities are classic sufferers of episodic acute stress. Traumatic stress is the result of massive acute stress, PTSD, for example.

Chronic stress, on the other hand, lingers and is often a result of boredom and stagnation, as well as prolonged negative circumstances such as a bad job or relationship, chronic poverty or unemployment. Symptoms might include diabetes, immune system suppression, even cancer.

CHANGE AND STRESS

We can be overstressed when there are too many demands on us, and we can be understressed when there is nothing to do and we feel like we aren't getting anywhere. The more major life changes that have occurred in your life during the past couple of years, the greater the chances of your becoming physically or emotionally ill (Holmes and Rahe 1967).

Alvin Toffler wrote a best seller, *Future Shock* (1970) which sets out the idea that technology produces such rapid change that people feel unable to keep up with the accelerating flow of information and choices. We are in a mobile society with few permanent relationships. Today almost everything is disposable, even our jobs and friends. We give them up and move on. Technology and the tendency to favour cheap labour threaten our jobs. On the other hand, an equal amount of stress or frustration is caused by changes being made too slowly rather than too fast, like racial prejudice, changes we'd like to make at work but can't, or the slow driver in front of us holding us up.

Siegelman (1983) and others speculate that change is upsetting because we are leaving a part of our selves behind. Any change involves a loss of the known, a giving up of a reality that has given meaning to our lives. We are also afraid we won't get the things we want after the change is made. Siegelman also believes that there is an opposite force to the resistance to change. It is natural to seek change, to master new challenges, explore the unknown and to test ourselves.

THE ROLE OF STRESS ON HEALTH

Chronic stress can be the result of repeated rounds of acute stress (episodic acute stress) or a life condition such as a difficult job situation or chronic disease. The thought of threat, on a continual basis, sends the message to our systems that the stress response, our survival mechanisms of fight-or-flight, need to be continually activated. In the fight-or-flight response of the sympathetic nervous system to threatening or harmful events, energy is diverted from internal organs to the muscles, heart rate increases and the body is made ready for physical action and increased sensory performance. Energy cannot be diverted in both directions simultaneously, so when danger has been identified and the body makes a fight-or-flight response, the body suppresses the immune response temporarily in order to maximize the energy available to deal with the threat.

Many functions in the body turn off because they are not needed in the fight-or-flight response. Other functions in the body are activated to higher than normal levels. However, when we are not in danger, continued activation of the stress response is not necessary. The stress response causes imbalances throughout normally functioning systems in the body, and when we see these responses, especially over an extended period, we need to make some changes to redress the balance.

Having to deal with a health condition can cause us anxiety and stress. Looking at it the other way round, those with long-term psychological issues such as anxiety, depression or anger are likely to be more stressed, which in turn can weaken the immune system (Hales 2003).

There is a plethora of research showing the link between the immune system and stress. Kiecolt-Glaser *et al.* (2002) explore how psychological factors influence immune function and the importance of personal relationships, and detail a range of conditions which may show a psychological–immune-system link, including ageing, cardiovascular disease, osteoporosis, arthritis, type 2 diabetes and certain cancers.

The way stress affects the immune system is described by Wein (2009). He explains that stress produces a hormone in the body called cortisol. The brain recognizes cortisol as the 'fight or flight' hormone, and when it is produced other body functions are halted until the stressful situation has passed. This is the body's way of taking care of an immediate emergency. The immune system also receives signals to slow down while cortisol does its job. However, with chronic stress the immune system stays in low gear, leaving the body vulnerable to infection and disease. Common illnesses brought on or worsened by stress are cardiovascular disease, digestive problems, skin conditions and poor memory function.

The effects of a compromised immune system are far-reaching including everything from susceptibility to the common cold to the rate of wound healing; it is even linked with breast cancer development. In research on women with metastatic breast cancer, psychiatrist David Spiegel found that stress hormones played a role in the progression of breast cancer (2010). The average survival time of women with normal cortisol patterns was significantly longer than that of women whose cortisol levels remained high throughout the day (an indicator of stress).

Long-term, chronic stress not only increases the risk of cardiovascular disease and compromises the immune system; the American Institute of Stress issued this statement about the long-term effects of stress:

> Many of these effects are due to increased sympathetic nervous system activity and an outpouring of adrenaline, cortisol, and other stress-related hormones. Certain types of chronic and more insidious stress due to loneliness, poverty, bereavement, depression and frustration due to discrimination are associated with impaired immune system resistance to viral linked disorders ranging from the common cold and herpes to AIDS and cancer. Stress can have effects on other hormones, brain neurotransmitters, additional small chemical messengers elsewhere, prostaglandins, as well as crucial enzyme systems, and metabolic activities that are still unknown. Research in these areas may help to explain how stress can contribute to depression, anxiety, and its diverse effects on the gastrointestinal tract, skin and other organs. (American Institute of Stress 2010)

All of the following disease conditions have been shown to have a stress component: abnormal heartbeat, alcoholism, asthma, chronic fatigue, chronic tension headaches, heart disease, depression, erectile dysfunction, skin disorders, high blood pressure, fertility, fibromyalgia, insomnia, IBS, menstrual difficulties, MS and ulcerative colitis.

In his book, *Mind as Healer, Mind as Slayer*, Kenneth Pelletier (1977, p.76) stated, 'Generalized, and unabated stress places a person in a state of disequilibrium, which increases his susceptibility to a wide range of diseases and disorders'. Research shows that stress alone will not cause illness. How a person reacts to stress is the critical factor which determines whether the outcome is positive or negative. The individual's way of viewing the events in life will determine the impact of stress.

Mindbody solutions

As we saw earlier in this module, there is a range of mindbody solutions. The interventions which are particularly useful to integrate into a wellness coaching practice include: biofeedback, prayer, flower essences, meditation, yoga, mood food, visualization and imagery, autogenic training, tai chi, creative therapies such as drama therapy, music and sand play, progressive muscle relaxation (PMR), breathing techniques, chi qong, art, exercise, hypnotherapy and self-hypnosis, journalling and mindfulness.

Integrating limiting client mindsets

Why is it that when two people are exposed to identical stressors, one experiences distressing physiological or psychological symptoms while the other comes through in a positive and healthy manner? How did this person manage to stay healthy? Research indicates that personality may be a key determinant in how well we are able to resist the negative influences of stress.

We see how our bodily systems can influence our mindset and visa versa. Let's stay with the mindset idea and see how it might affect a wellness coaching client.

Limited mindsets

What we think and believe influences our emotional state and consequently our behaviours. These are some of the limiting mindsets clients can come to therapy and wellness coaching with:

- The child mindset: I want to be looked after – You do it – Someone else will do it (for me) – I'll be taken care of now – The healthcare professional must know all (and it must be right) – Someone else will have the answer – Being ill gets me attention – I'll have to grow up – I am unsafe – I don't know how to care for myself – It will hurt – I want a magic wand.

- The escapist mindset: I'll have to do something I don't want to do if I get better – I can avoid doing [something I don't want to do].

- The denial mindset: It's not happening to me – I'll eat/drink/smoke/work my way through it – It's easier to be ill than feel anger, etc.

- The guilty mindset: It's my fault I'm ill – I've failed because I'm ill – I'm weak because I'm ill – I'm not perfect because I'm ill – I must be a bad person or have done something wrong.

- The angry mindset: The medical profession don't know anything – It's their fault – He/she will be under my control if I'm ill.

- The stoic mindset: I mustn't be ill (e.g. Who will look after the family?) – I must keep going – I don't need any help – Treatment is for weak people – I mustn't be helpless/dependent – I've got permission to be ill now.

- The victim mindset: I can't cope – It's all too much for me – I don't understand – Why has this happened to me? – No one really cares abut me, so why should I? – I'm alone so why should I care? – Nobody cares – I'm going to die – It's all over – There's no point – I can't change anything – I'll lose everything – Nothing can change this disease/condition – There's nothing left – I can't do anything to change this – No one can do anything for me – There's no cure – I've got no choice – I won't get any better – I've got nothing to get better for – I deserve to be ill – It's not fair – I don't deserve wellness – It's winter and everyone's ill – I'll get it wrong.

Where do these mindsets come from? If we consider nature and nurture influences, these mindsets may come from the client's core personality as well as learned responses from parents or beliefs arising from life experiences. These potentially limiting mindsets can hold a client back from getting the most from wellness coaching.

How to help clients move past limited mindsets

As wellness coaches, we have the opportunity to work with clients to help them move past their limited mindsets so that they can achieve their wellness goals.

CHALLENGE THE CLIENT'S MINDSET WITH COMPASSION

However frustrated you may feel in response to clients' apparent negativity or unwillingness to change, be compassionate. They have come to you for help and as a wellness coach (and therapist); we know how clients can hide their needs behind fear and resistance. Balance compassion with practical realism. Most clients are fearful of the implications of not being healthy or of the changes that may need to be made. Consider how your clients may be feeling, what their mindset may be and how you can help them come from a better place.

FACILITATE THE CLIENT MOVING INTO SELF-RESPONSIBILITY

Clients are more likely to change when they take responsibility. So often, they come wanting us to do the work or wave the magic wand. They have the wand. We can help them find it. Once a client picks up self-responsibility and moves from child to adult, we can work with the client to produce more effective results. To facilitate moving clients into self-responsibility, ask them questions, help them find stability zones in the midst of change, treat them like adults, coach them in skills which empower to them and show them the pay-offs for taking responsibility. Responsibility is not about guilt or blame but about empowerment. When clients are empowered through taking responsibility, they have more ability to act creatively.

FACILITATE THE CLIENT IN MANAGING CHANGE AND TRANSITION

Wellness coaching is about change, moving from one state of being or doing to another. Resistant clients often fear a perceived loss or unwanted gain from the change. By coaching clients in change management, you will be helping to reassure them they can move forward. Help clients to see their condition as an opportunity for change. However your clients may choose to see wellness, and whichever routes they want to take, your role is to facilitate their journey. Change becomes opportunity.

DISPLACING

Instead of getting to grips with the issue at hand, some clients complain about physical problems rather than talk about emotional pain. Or they may deal with emotional pain by turning to drink, drugs, food or another addiction. If exploring displacement activities doesn't help clients, they may not be coaching-ready.

BOUNDARIES

Only today I was talking with an art therapist about how it took her forever to move a client out of the door at the end of her session. Some clients have little sense of boundaries. They come too early or late, or they stay stuck to the chair at the end of the session and can only be moved with a psychological crowbar. Other ways clients may be not be respectful of boundaries is the persistent inclusion of inappropriate subjects or asking you personal questions. As the wellness coach, it is your responsibility to hold the boundary. If clients keep coming too early or late, challenge them. Warn them when a session is coming to an end. End it on time. If necessary, get up and go to the door. Use firm but positive body language to end the session. If clients keep including inappropriate subject matter, point it out and move the subject on. If they ask you personal questions, answer very generally and move on. If necessary, you may need to challenge their behaviour. If you feel uncomfortable, you can end the session, refuse to see them again or refer them on. Always talk through your client concerns with your supervisor.

FACILITATE THE CLIENT IN MANAGING UNCERTAINTY

All too often with health-related issues, there is uncertainty. Will it work? Will it last? How will it manifest? What will change as a result? There are many questions and not always a certain answer. Managing uncertainty sounds like a contradiction, but it is possible to manage by reducing risks. Uncertainty and the need to take risks are an inherent part of any new wellness opportunity. You can help your clients gain the confidence they need to explore new opportunities.

COACH THE CLIENT IN ASSERTIVE BEHAVIOUR

Assertiveness may arise in relation to a client and a healthcare professional such as a GP or consultant. Or it might be that the client needs to set boundaries with work colleagues or in personal relationships. If you are in doubt as a wellness coach how to coach someone in assertiveness skills, go on a short course yourself as a participant.

MOTIVATE THE CLIENT

If clients aren't motivated to making wellness changes, very little will change for them. Motivation can arise from a perceived reward, for example 'I'll feel better', or penalty, 'If I don't do this, I won't be able to do my job well and I might get the sack'. Find out what motivates your clients and keep reminding them. You can tell if motivation is low or misplaced because the client won't engage in the wellness coaching process.

INSPIRE FAITH AND HOPE

What is the difference between these two states? When we lose faith, we falter. We are lost in a void where there seems to be no way through, and we feel weak. Faith seems to come of a core inner knowledge and gives strength, power and trust.

Hopelessness is heavy; body, mind and spirit are weary. Hope comes from our essence, the core – maybe the spirit. It's a place where light shows and ripples out to the mind with strength to give courage and faith.

As wellness coaches, we have the opportunity to inspire our clients to find their way to hope and faith and help clients use these states to motivate themselves. We might do this through philosophical, spiritual or religious means. Take whatever pathway the client needs to explore.

RAISE SELF-ESTEEM

Here are five ways you can coach your clients to improve their self-esteem:

- Help your clients get past the need to be perfect. Aiming for perfection in life is a lost cause because it means different things to different people. Nobody is perfect in the eyes of everyone else, so by trying to be perfect you set yourself up for disappointment and failure. Instead, coach your clients to achieve wellness goals.

- Help your clients improve their self confidence by doing things that make them feel good, like accomplishing something.

- Coach your clients in how to appreciate themselves. Everyone has strengths, weaknesses, habits and principles that define who they are. Coach your clients in focusing on the qualities about themselves they like, and less on the ones that they dislike.

- Coach your clients in facing their fears and learning from their failures. When things don't go the way they would like it to, there is something to be learned from that, which can be applied next time they are in a similar situation.

- Coach your clients in how to reward themselves when they succeed.

BUILD RAPPORT FOR THE CLIENT TO BE OPEN

Building rapport is a key component in allowing clients to trust enough to risk opening themselves up. It isn't only to us that they are opening up, but, more important, to themselves. We might be the first person to hear and witness a client's hopes and fears. When clients understand that we are there for them in a non-judgemental way, the celebration is in seeing their courage come out.

USE CREATIVE AND LATERAL APPROACHES

Come from a place of creativity when working with clients. Speak their language (it builds rapport) and gently ease back their boundaries of self-knowledge and action. Create your toolbox of wellness coaching techniques and encourage clients to create theirs.

ENCOURAGE THE CLIENT TO BECOME INFORMED

The wellness coaching process is non-directive, and part of our work is to encourage clients to become informed through their own efforts. This can happen as part of negotiated tasks between sessions and during the session.

> ### Inside tip
>
> When I start to work with a student who wants to become a coach, the two most common mindsets are that the coach has to know everything, and to provide solutions for the client.
>
> Both mindsets are wrong. No one can know everything. A wellness coach does need to know how to facilitate clients on their journey of becoming informed, and how clients can use that information. There is a difference between a client who genuinely doesn't know and a client who can't be bothered. If clients truly don't know, their body language will be open and positive if a little befuddled. We can help these clients along. If clients can't be bothered, their body language will give it away. Then we challenge them more – or confront their behaviour!
>
> The client has the solutions…or at least the nugget of solutions. We facilitate the journey of self-discovery. We don't spoon-feed the client.

Show clients how they can integrate healthcare modalities. There are a thousand tools a client to use in his wellness programme with you. As well as any work he may do with you therapeutically or through wellness coaching, he may also have other methods and people to help him in other ways. Part of his wellness coaching is to integrate a network of healthcare modalities.

EXPLORE PHILOSOPHICAL/SPIRITUAL/RELIGIOUS PATHWAYS

Many spiritual, religious or philosophical pathways can weave together to form the basis of wellness. These pathways are the canvas, the groundwork upon which we can build more practical structures. Not every client wants to explore these pathways, yet the opportunity should always be placed before them.

COACH THE CLIENT IN SELF-NOURISHMENT

As therapists, we are aware that people can come for counselling or complementary therapy not only because they have immediate issues, but because they have a need for nourishment from another. We may provide a safe space for the client to explore and develop and this act in itself is nourishing. However, it is important as wellness coaches to encourage self-nourishment in our clients.

COACH THE CLIENT IN MINDFULNESS

Mindfulness is about living in the now. Not sinking in past guilt or future fear, but standing firm in the now of the moment. Now is the point of healing, of wellness.

HELP THE CLIENT REDEFINE WHAT HEALING IS

Many clients come to us with expectations of what healing is. Some will want their symptoms to lessen or go away. Others want reassurance. Some expect us to collude with them in their denial or fantasies. Part of our work as wellness coaches is to offer new ways for defining healing.

HELP THE CLIENT LET GO

It may be that clients need to let of their expectations of what wellness, health or healing is in order to move on. It may be that clients need to identify and let go of faulty mindsets about something, for example how it's not feminine for women to be angry. It may be that clients need to let go of a particular behaviour, for example eating high-fat food.

HELP THE CLIENT FIND MEANING

I hesitated at this one, pondering on whether *motivation* is the same as *meaning*. The motivation for me to lower my cholesterol is to increase my heart wellness, especially as heart disease runs in my family. To 'find meaning' for me isn't connected to a practical outcome but has something of an intrinsic essence, or slant. For example, writing is intrinsic for me. It is a tool for my intrinsic wellness (although there was a practical outcome when I kept a journal throughout my breast cancer experience). Helping your clients find meaning will open up their wellness opportunities.

WORKING WITH UNCOMMITTED CLIENTS

Lack of commitment can be a challenging problem in the coaching setting. Normally, clients with little or no commitment have specific agendas which justify their attendance, such as having a partner who wants the client to attend wellness coaching to lose weight. The client is there to please her partner (whether she wants to or not is another matter). Framing and reframing are good tactics to remodel the way the client perceives the coaching relationship in order to move into a collaborative approach – or to end it if that is what she wants. Creating goals and structuring will motivate clients to go through the necessary stages for change, collect the rewards, and move on with their life.

HELP THE CLIENT BE POSITIVE AND REALISTIC

Clients may present for wellness coaching with unrealistic expectations. Your work as a wellness coach is to co-create realistic goals. These goals may not always be what clients want and their responses might not be very positive, and therefore they may not be too motivated. At this time, you need to coach them in other ways of looking at their redefined goals. Ways in which they could view them as positive. This in turn, will increase their motivation.

HELP CLIENTS TO SEE THEIR CONDITIONS AND HEALING AS A PATH OF SELF-DISCOVERY

Not all clients can or want to see their wellness programme as a means of self-discovery. Some will want to; others may not be able to. When clients can see their personal growth through their condition, they gain insight and this adds to their motivation. This isn't always easy, especially with debilitating or progressive conditions or with lifestyle changes that seem all-consuming.

HELP THE CLIENT TO FORGIVE THEMSELVES

Self-forgiveness can sound crass when clients are faced with health conditions. What I mean here is not beating yourself up if you can't quite achieve a wellness goal, but to learn from the experience, identify what went well and what realistically can be changed.

There could also be elements of self-dislike if clients believe they're a failure if they get ill or can't complete an agreed task. At these times, exploring faulty thinking and beliefs through cognitive behavioural coaching might be useful.

WORKING WITH A DEMANDING CLIENT

Demanding clients normally believe that the wellness coach will provide answers to their problems. They will come to coaching without much resolve to act upon their current situation, and will normally create unrealistic expectations regarding the coaching relationship and the coach. Encouraging accountability, managing expectations and establishing well-planned goals is a good approach. The client should be encouraged to realize that change can only occur from within. Using a solution-focused approach to empower and encourage the client may be the key for deriving motivation.

ALLOW THE CLIENT TO EXPRESS VULNERABILITY

If a client is dealing with health issues or looking to making life changes to improve life (or transition) quality, she is in a vulnerable place. Opening up to herself and you takes trust, courage and honesty. Providing a safe space and building rapport will allow clients to express their vulnerability.

ALLOW THE CLIENT TO GRIEVE

With progressive or terminal illness, there can be much to grieve through. Many may need to come to terms with a disability. Allow time for grieving.

> ### Inside tip
>
> I facilitated several writing groups for women going through the breast cancer journey. We explored issues around loss – for example, loss of hair, loss of perceived perfect health, loss of freedom, loss of a breast, loss of a relationship, etc. Allowing time for writing and verbal sharing helped many women along their journey of grieving and, in turn, healing.

SUPPORT CLIENTS AS THEY MOVE THROUGH FEAR

There can be much to fear when engaging in wellness coaching. Indeed, fear may be the motivator for a client's coming to see you. It is important to hear your client's fear and to balance realism with reassurance.

WHAT IS THE CLIENT TRYING TO EXPRESS?

Sometimes physical symptoms are a symbolic physical expression of what a client is unable to express – for example an anniversary illness. Unexpressed thoughts and feelings can block the flow of energy throughout the subtle and physical body, thereby depressing the immune system and creating disease.

LEARNED RESPONSES

What impact have clients' conditioning had on their expectations of health and illness? For example, is there a parent in your client's background who has always been 'needy'? Is this part of the reason your client doesn't know how to look after himself? How do the client's past experiences impact his current attitude towards wellness and healing?

WORKING WITH A SCEPTICAL CLIENT

You may find yourself working with clients who come to wellness coaching either to please someone else or as a last resort. They will be sceptical about the process, and may not acknowledge any need to change. It is important for the coach to gain respect from the client and use that respect to establish trust. One of the most common strategies to gain respect and create responsiveness from the client is to outline the process of wellness coaching, what she is there for, the structure of the relationship, the rights and responsibilities of the client and what might be the expected positive outcomes. Solution-focused strategies are a good way to create a sense of accountability and need for change.

INTEGRATING SHADOW AND LIGHT

Much of our time is spent running or hiding from our selves, looking outside, everywhere and anywhere apart from where the truth is. We may not like parts of our nature, but they are still part of our wholeness. When we see, understand and accept this, we can reclaim the dark and transmute it into light and energy. Therefore every experience we have takes us towards a deepening consciousness.

EXPLORE THE CLIENT'S EXPECTATIONS

What do clients expect of themselves in the wellness coaching process? Or are they trying to fulfill someone else's expectations of their wellness?

ENCOURAGE AWARENESS

Life (and therefore energy) occurs simultaneously on three levels: physical, mental/emotional and spiritual. Awareness needs to occur on all levels. Awareness is a profound inner journeying and requires exploring all that stands between self and essence, such as beliefs about worth, sickness and health.

No one person, wellness coach or therapist, has the monopoly on the truth. We experience different realities. What got us here today may not work for us tomorrow. What works for you may not work for me because we have different internal and external realities. As Hippocrates said, 'The natural healing force within each one of us is the greatest force in getting well'.

An integrated wellness coaching example

To *integrate* means to form or unit into a whole. When applied to wellness coaching, we co-creating an integrated wellness plan with the client. Take the example in Figure 2.3 of a client with high blood pressure.

The client comes to you wanting to reduce or come off his blood pressure medication. Let's assume with a positive mind frame that he wants to be proactive with his wellness programme and is willing to explore his lifestyle and mindset. His dietary habits are not healthy and he is overweight, his activity levels low and his stress levels high.

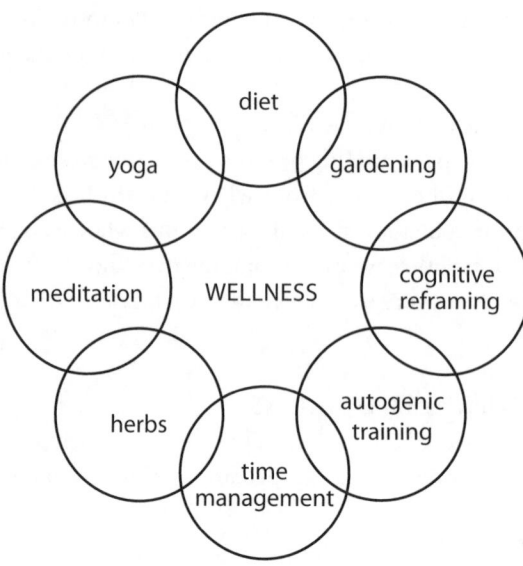

Figure 2.3 An integrated wellness coaching plan for a client with high blood pressure

Cognitive coaching occurs in the sessions to understand the mindsets which contribute to inappropriate behaviour. Time-management coaching is given. He needs coaching in client-centred activities such as meditation, yoga and autogenic training which he can then practise on a regular basis, building them into his lifestyle. Nutritional coaching can lead to weight-reducing eating and drinking habits outside of the coaching room. Herbal supplementation under the guidance of a nutritionist or herbalist is built-in. Gardening is a self-chosen activity which can also be creative and relaxing. The client's GP is informed of the wellness coaching plan. The client is coached in monitoring his own blood pressure with regular check-ins with you and the GP. In time, medication is reduced, leading to the possibility of coming off the medication altogether. Regular, self-monitored blood pressure check-ups are necessary with the understanding that should the blood pressure rise above a certain point, either a wellness coach or the GP is consulted.

CPD task sheet

This is your Continuing Professional Development (CPD) task sheet which summarizes key module points and offers you the opportunity to engage with tasks to deepen your learning.

Module summary

- Physical and psychological wellness is influenced by social interactions, environmental influences, work practices and spiritual beliefs.

- Both client and wellness coach bring eclectic mindsets into the sessions.

- Being client-centred is important to the wellness coaching process.

- Be mindful of the boundaries between counselling and coaching.

- Engage in a co-creative process with the wellness coaching client.

- Wellness coaches need to straddle the curative and preventative boundary.

- Know when and how to integrate therapies into wellness coaching.

- Understand the building blocks of the mindbody and stress link and how to integrate them into the wellness coaching dynamics.

- Identify and integrate client mindsets towards wellness and health.

Your tasks

1. Consider your wellness from physical, psychological, social, environmental, work and spiritual perspectives.

2. What mindsets around wellness do you have? What are the differences between your personal and professional mindsets, if any?

3. How client-centred are you?

4. Consider the boundaries between counselling and coaching. If you are a counsellor, reflect on the boundary issue for you. If you are not a counsellor, how will you keep the boundaries or become more informed or skilled?

5. Practise the co-creative process with a colleague or friend.

6. Are you more curative- or preventative-inclined in your healthcare services?

7. Research the mindbody connection further.

8. Reflect upon past and current clients and the varying mindsets they have presented with towards their healing process.

Key Issues with Wellness Coaching

By the end of the module, you will have explored:

- Differences between coaching, counselling and mentoring
- Core coaching competencies
- How people learn
- Coaching models
- The importance of client motivation
- The importance of managing change
- Wellness coaching networks

Differences between coaching, counselling and mentoring

As healthcare professionals, we aim for an integrated wellness coaching model. As we do this, it is important to understand the differences between the principles of coaching, counselling and mentoring. Within the wellness coaching role, it is easy to slide from one to the other.

Coaching principles

The wellness coach provides feedback on strengths and weaknesses and is patient, nurturing, evocative, cathartic, catalytic and challenging. The coach can appropriately identify important unfinished emotional business which hampers client performance and is aware of how thoughts and emotional reactions can lead to problematic behaviours.

Wellness coaches need to develop the ability to be fully conscious in the creation of a relationship with the client, employing a style that is open and spontaneous. They need to be present and flexible during the coaching process and see a variety of ways to work with clients, choosing in the moment, what is most effective. They need to be able to confidently shift perspectives and experiment with new possibilities for action. Wellness coaches need to demonstrate confidence in working with strong emotions, and show self-management in order not to be enmeshed by the client's emotions. In addition, they need to be able to use humour effectively to create lightness and energy and to access their intuitive processes.

Wellness coaching has a specific focus on improving wellness across a range of lifestyle issues. It is about learning and development and has a specific agenda of identified attainable and measurable goals. Wellness coaching is normally short term, with each session lasting between 45 minutes and 2 hours. It is performance-related, action- and outcome-orientated, with results being attained fairly quickly. Wellness coaching:

- may also involve outside reference
- has structured sessions and can take place anywhere
- is present and future orientated
- is accountability focused and asks: how – what – when and why?
- is co-creative and non-directive
- assumes that the individual is psychologically well and does not require a clinical intervention
- will explore the past in relation to the present and future goals
- fine tunes and develops skills.

Counselling principles

The counsellor leads clients towards self-directed actions to achieve their goals and is patient, nurturing, evocative, parenting and cathartic. Counselling tends to take place in a therapeutic or clinical environment and may be short or long term, each session lasting 50–60 minutes. It is a slow process and explores psychosocial issues through discussion in order to increase understanding or develop greater self-awareness. Counselling:

- seeks to understand and resolve the past through deep and sometimes intense emotional experiences
- is based on feelings and asks why, seeking improvement of emotional states
- can be medically or clinically related.

Mentoring principles

The mentor is a role model of expertise and experience and an advocate for the mentee to support his growth and development. Mentoring offers an ongoing long-term relationship and is key to professional development. It is informal, broad and opens doors through sharing knowledge. The technique focuses on individual development and utilizes coaching strategies.

Core coaching competencies

Professional coaches provide an ongoing partnership designed to help clients produce fulfilling results in their personal and professional lives. Coaches help people improve their performances and enhance the quality of their lives.

The following 11 core coaching competencies were developed to support greater understanding about the skills and approaches used within today's coaching profession as defined by the International Coach Federation (ICF) (2010) (used with permission).

A. Setting the foundation

1. **Meeting Ethical Guidelines and Professional Standards** – Understanding of coaching ethics and standards and ability to apply them appropriately in all coaching situations

   a. Understands and exhibits in own behaviors the ICF Standards of Conduct (see list),

   b. Understands and follows all ICF Ethical Guidelines (see list),

   c. Clearly communicates the distinctions between coaching, consulting, psychotherapy and other support professions,

   d. Refers client to another support professional as needed, knowing when this is needed and the available resources.

2. **Establishing the Coaching Agreement** – Ability to understand what is required in the specific coaching interaction and to come to agreement with the prospective and new client about the coaching process and relationship

   a. Understands and effectively discusses with the client the guidelines and specific parameters of the coaching relationship (e.g., logistics, fees, scheduling, inclusion of others if appropriate),

   b. Reaches agreement about what is appropriate in the relationship and what is not, what is and is not being offered, and about the client's and coach's responsibilities,

   c. Determines whether there is an effective match between his/her coaching method and the needs of the prospective client.

B. Co-creating the relationship

1. **Establishing Trust and Intimacy with the Client** – Ability to create a safe, supportive environment that produces ongoing mutual respect and trust

   a. Shows genuine concern for the client's welfare and future,

   b. Continuously demonstrates personal integrity, honesty and sincerity,

   c. Establishes clear agreements and keeps promises,

   d. Demonstrates respect for client's perceptions, learning style, personal being,

   e. Provides ongoing support for and champions new behaviors and actions, including those involving risk taking and fear of failure,

   f. Asks permission to coach client in sensitive, new areas.

2. **Coaching Presence** – Ability to be fully conscious and create spontaneous relationship with the client, employing a style that is open, flexible and confident

   a. Is present and flexible during the coaching process, dancing in the moment,

   b. Accesses own intuition and trusts one's inner knowing – 'goes with the gut',

   c. Is open to not knowing and takes risks,

   d. Sees many ways to work with the client, and chooses in the moment what is most effective,

   e. Uses humor effectively to create lightness and energy,

   f. Confidently shifts perspectives and experiments with new possibilities for own action,

   g. Demonstrates confidence in working with strong emotions, and can self-manage and not be overpowered or enmeshed by client's emotions.

C. Communicating effectively

1. **Active Listening** – Ability to focus completely on what the client is saying and is not saying, to understand the meaning of what is said in the context of the client's desires, and to support client self-expression

   a. Attends to the client and the client's agenda, and not to the coach's agenda for the client,

b. Hears the client's concerns, goals, values and beliefs about what is and is not possible,

c. Distinguishes between the words, the tone of voice, and the body language,

d. Summarizes, paraphrases, reiterates, mirrors back what client has said to ensure clarity and understanding,

e. Encourages, accepts, explores and reinforces the client's expression of feelings, perceptions, concerns, beliefs, suggestions, etc.,

f. Integrates and builds on client's ideas and suggestions,

g. 'Bottom-lines' or understands the essence of the client's communication and helps the client get there rather than engaging in long descriptive stories,

h. Allows the client to vent or 'clear' the situation without judgment or attachment in order to move on to next steps.

2. **Powerful Questioning** – Ability to ask questions that reveal the information needed for maximum benefit to the coaching relationship and the client

a. Asks questions that reflect active listening and an understanding of the client's perspective,

b. Asks questions that evoke discovery, insight, commitment or action (e.g., those that challenge the client's assumptions),

c. Asks open-ended questions that create greater clarity, possibility or new learning,

d. Asks questions that move the client towards what they desire, not questions that ask for the client to justify or look backwards.

3. **Direct Communication** – Ability to communicate effectively during coaching sessions, and to use language that has the greatest positive impact on the client

a. Is clear, articulate and direct in sharing and providing feedback,

b. Reframes and articulates to help the client understand from another perspective what he/she wants or is uncertain about,

c. Clearly states coaching objectives, meeting agenda, purpose of techniques or exercises,

d. Uses language appropriate and respectful to the client (e.g., non-sexist, non-racist, non-technical, non-jargon),

e. Uses metaphor and analogy to help to illustrate a point or paint a verbal picture.

D. Facilitating learning and results

1. **Creating Awareness** – Ability to integrate and accurately evaluate multiple sources of information, and to make interpretations that help the client to gain awareness and thereby achieve agreed-upon results

   a. Goes beyond what is said in assessing client's concerns, not getting hooked by the client's description,

   b. Invokes inquiry for greater understanding, awareness and clarity,

   c. Identifies for the client his/her underlying concerns, typical and fixed ways of perceiving himself/herself and the world, differences between the facts and the interpretation, disparities between thoughts, feelings and action,

   d. Helps clients to discover for themselves the new thoughts, beliefs, perceptions, emotions, moods, etc. that strengthen their ability to take action and achieve what is important to them,

   e. Communicates broader perspectives to clients and inspires commitment to shift their viewpoints and find new possibilities for action,

   f. Helps clients to see the different, interrelated factors that affect them and their behaviors (e.g., thoughts, emotions, body, background),

   g. Expresses insights to clients in ways that are useful and meaningful for the client,

   h. Identifies major strengths vs. major areas for learning and growth, and what is most important to address during coaching,

   i. Asks the client to distinguish between trivial and significant issues, situational vs. recurring behaviors, when detecting a separation between what is being stated and what is being done.

2. **Designing Actions** – Ability to create with the client opportunities for ongoing learning, during coaching and in work/life situations, and for taking new actions that will most effectively lead to agreed-upon coaching results

   a. Brainstorms and assists the client to define actions that will enable the client to demonstrate, practice and deepen new learning,

   b. Helps the client to focus on and systematically explore specific concerns and opportunities that are central to agreed-upon coaching goals,

   c. Engages the client to explore alternative ideas and solutions, to evaluate options, and to make related decisions,

    d. Promotes active experimentation and self-discovery, where the client applies what has been discussed and learned during sessions immediately afterwards in his/her work or life setting,

    e. Celebrates client successes and capabilities for future growth,

    f. Challenges client's assumptions and perspectives to provoke new ideas and find new possibilities for action,

    g. Advocates or brings forward points of view that are aligned with client goals and, without attachment, engages the client to consider them,

    h. Helps the client 'Do It Now' during the coaching session, providing immediate support,

    i. Encourages stretches and challenges but also a comfortable pace of learning.

3. **Planning and Goal Setting** – Ability to develop and maintain an effective coaching plan with the client

    a. Consolidates collected information and establishes a coaching plan and development goals with the client that address concerns and major areas for learning and development,

    b. Creates a plan with results that are attainable, measurable, specific and have target dates,

    c. Makes plan adjustments as warranted by the coaching process and by changes in the situation,

    d. Helps the client identify and access different resources for learning (e.g., books, other professionals),

    e. Identifies and targets early successes that are important to the client.

4. **Managing Progress and Accountability** – Ability to hold attention on what is important for the client, and to leave responsibility with the client to take action

    a. Clearly requests of the client actions that will move the client towards their stated goals,

    b. Demonstrates follow through by asking the client about those actions that the client committed to during the previous session(s),

    c. Acknowledges the client for what they have done, not done, learned or become aware of since the previous coaching session(s),

d. Effectively prepares, organizes and reviews with client information obtained during sessions,

e. Keeps the client on track between sessions by holding attention on the coaching plan and outcomes, agreed-upon courses of action, and topics for future session(s),

f. Focuses on the coaching plan but is also open to adjusting behaviors and actions based on the coaching process and shifts in direction during sessions,

g. Is able to move back and forth between the big picture of where the client is heading, setting a context for what is being discussed and where the client wishes to go,

h. Promotes client's self-discipline and holds the client accountable for what they say they are going to do, for the results of an intended action, or for a specific plan with related time frames,

i. Develops the client's ability to make decisions, address key concerns, and develop himself/herself (to get feedback, to determine priorities and set the pace of learning, to reflect on and learn from experiences),

j. Positively confronts the client with the fact that he/she did not take agreed-upon actions.

How people learn

Much of what your client will achieve in her wellness programme will depend how she learns. By identifying your client's preferred style, you can apply this methodology when coaching wellness. If you can utilize your client's natural style, her progress will be easier and quicker. Here are a number of learning approaches:

Anthony Gregorc's model

Anthony F. Gregorc and Kathleen A. Butler (Gregorc 1984) organized a model describing how the mind works. This model is based on the existence of perceptions and our evaluation of the world. These perceptions in turn are the foundation of our specific learning styles.

In this model, there are two perceptual qualities: concrete and abstract. Concrete perceptions involve registering information through the five senses, while abstract perceptions involve the understanding of ideas, qualities and concepts which cannot be seen.

There are also two ordering abilities: random and sequential. The sequential ordering ability involves the organization of information in a linear, logical way;

random involves the organization of information in chunks and in no specific order.

Both of the perceptual qualities and both of the ordering abilities are present in each individual, but some qualities and ordering abilities are more dominant within certain individuals. There are four combinations of perceptual qualities and ordering abilities based on dominance:

- Concrete Sequential
- Abstract Random
- Abstract Sequential
- Concrete Random.

Individuals with different combinations learn in different ways. They have different strengths, different things make sense to them, different things are difficult for them and they ask different questions throughout the learning process.

Fleming's VAK/VARK model

One of the most common and widely-used categorizations of the various types of learning styles is Neil Fleming's VARK model (Fleming and Mills 1992) which expanded upon earlier VAK models:

- Visual learners have a preference for seeing and think in pictures. (Use visual aids such as diagrams and handouts, leave white space in handouts for note-taking, invite questions, use flipcharts, supplement textual information with illustrations, have the learners envision the topic or have them act out the subject matter.)

- Auditory learners best learn through listening. (Use discussions, CDs, the Socratic method of talking by questioning learners to draw as much information from them as possible and then filling in the gaps with your expertise, include auditory activities like brainstorming, leave plenty of time to debrief activities, ask your client what questions they have and work on developing a dialogue between yourself and the client.)

- Reading/writing-preference learners.

- Kinesthetic or tactile learners prefer to learn via experience, moving and doing. (Use activities that get them, use coloured markers to emphasize key points on flipcharts or whiteboards, give frequent stretch breaks, guide learners through a visualization of complex tasks.)

Learners can also use the model to identify their preferred learning style and maximize their experience by focusing on what benefits them the most.

David Kolb's learning styles model and experiential learning theory

David Kolb, Professor of Organizational Behaviour at Case Western Reserve University, is credited with launching the learning styles movement in the early 1970s and published his learning styles model in 1984. He sets out four distinct learning styles which are based on a four-stage learning cycle. The David Kolb styles model is based on the experiential learning theory (ELT), as explained in his book *Experiential Learning: Experience as the Source of Learning and Development* (1984). The ELT outlines two related models of grasping experience: concrete experience and abstract conceptualization, as well as two related approaches towards transforming experience: reflective observation and active experimentation. According to Kolb's model, the ideal learning process engages all four of these modes in response to situational demands. In order for learning to be effective, all four of these approaches must be incorporated. As individuals attempt to use all four approaches, however, they tend to develop strengths in one experience-grasping approach and one experience-transforming approach. The resulting learning styles are combinations of the individual's preferred approaches. These learning styles are as follows.

- Converger: These learners are characterized by abstract conceptualization and active experimentation. They are good at making practical applications of ideas and using deductive reasoning to solve problems.

- Diverger: These learners tend towards concrete experience and reflective observation. They are imaginative and are good at coming up with ideas and seeing things from different perspectives.

- Assimilator: These learners are characterized by abstract conceptualization and reflective observation. They are capable of creating theoretical models by means of inductive reasoning.

- Accommodator: These learners use concrete experience and active experimentation. They are good at actively engaging with the world and actually doing things instead of merely reading about and studying them.

Kolb's model gave rise to the Learning Style Inventory, an assessment method used to determine an individual's learning style. An individual may exhibit a preference for one of the four styles – Accommodating, Converging, Diverging and Assimilating – depending on his approach to learning via the experiential learning theory model.

Honey and Mumford Learning Styles Questionnaire

In the mid 1970s, Peter Honey and Alan Mumford adapted David Kolb's model for use with a population of middle and senior managers in business. They published their version of the model in *The Manual of Learning Styles* (1982) and *Using Your Learning Styles* (1983). Two adaptations were made to Kolb's experiential model. First, the stages in the cycle were renamed to accord with managerial experiences of decision-making and problem-solving. The Honey and Mumford stages are:

1. having an experience

2. reviewing the experience

3. concluding from the experience

4. planning the next steps.

Second, the styles were directly aligned to the stages in the cycle and named Activist, Reflector, Theorist and Pragmatist. These are assumed to be acquired preferences that are adaptable, either at will or through changed circumstances, rather than being fixed personality characteristics. The Honey and Mumford Learning Styles Questionnaire is a self-development tool. These learning styles are an indication only. It wouldn't be appropriate to button-hole clients in any one way. However, bear in mind how your client likes to learn and facilitate your sessions around those styles.

Coaching models

A coaching model is a framework; it does not tell you how to coach but is rather the underlying structure for your coaching.

The GROW model

The GROW model was developed in the UK by Sir John Whitmore and used extensively in coaching during the late 1980s and 1990s. It is described in a number of coaching books, including John Whitmore's book *Coaching for Performance: GROWing People, Performance and Purpose* (2009). GROW is an acronym for Goal, (current) Reality, Options and Will, which are seen as the four key elements of a coaching session.

GOAL

A session needs to have a goal. The goal should be as specific as possible and achievement needs to be measurable. Follow the SMART rule – make your goals specific, measurable, attainable, realistic and timely. Ask the following to identify the goal:

- What do you want to achieve?
- Why do you want to achieve it?
- Do you need to break down this goal into smaller goals?

REALITY

The second step is to determine what the current reality is in relation to your goal. This can be a key part of the wellness coaching session. By seeing clearly the situation rather than what was imagined, the resolution becomes obvious. Ask the following to clarify the reality:

- What is your current situation?
- What are the barriers at this moment? What's slowing you down?
- What have you tried so far that you could try differently?

OPTIONS

The third step is to understand your unique strengths which you can use to reach your goals. Ask:

- What makes you feel strong?
- What do you love to do?
- How can you have more of this?

WILL

The final step is the motivation for why you're doing what you're doing. This provides the will to make the journey. The *W* is often taken to stand for a number of other elements of a session, all of which are important. Myles Downey in his book *Effective Coaching* (2003) suggests it stands for 'Wrap-up'; others have it standing for What, Where, Why, When and How. But whatever is emphasized, the desired outcome from this stage is a commitment to action. Ask:

- What would reaching your goals do for you?
- What actions can you take right away?
- What will move you along when things are slow?

SUCCESS coaching model

THE MEANING

- **S**: Session planning
- **U**: Uplifting experiences
- **C**: Charting your course
- **C**: Creating opportunities
- **E**: Expectations and commitments
- **S**: Synergy
- **S**: Summary

SESSION PLANNING

This step, completed prior, will give structure to the session. You could ask clients: What actions will you commit to? What challenges have you faced since the previous session? What will be the focus for the next session? These clarifying questions allow you to keep the momentum going and also help your clients focus on what's important.

UPLIFTING EXPERIENCES

Most successful people build on their success. It's important to your clients' success to recall positive moments in life so they can continually build on them.

CHART YOUR COURSE

While you're working with your clients on topics that they've chosen, you'll be asking questions to help them move forward towards their goals.

CREATING OPPORTUNITIES

Where do your clients need to move forward? You're helping them understand what opportunities exist or how they can create ways to accomplish their goals.

EXPECTATIONS AND COMMITMENTS

What do your clients expect to achieve? Personal change requires a commitment to change and action.

SYNERGY

What is the energy between what your client has chosen to do and how she feels about doing it like? If it's not congruent, she's going to have a hard time changing. A big reason why people end up not doing what they've committed to do is because they don't really feel all good about doing it. This blocks energy, and energy influences many levels.

SUMMARY

What did the client get out of his wellness coaching? This step is a recap of what's been worked on during the session. If a client doesn't anchor his thoughts and ideas, he'll likely forget them as soon as he steps out the door. So make sure you're asking your client what he learned.

STEPPPA coaching model

Attributed to Angus McLeod, author of *Performance Coaching Toolkit* (McLeod and Thomas 2010), STEPPPA stands for:

- **S**ubject
- **T**arget Identification
- **E**motion
- **P**erception and Choice
- **P**lan
- **P**ace
- **A**dapt or Act

The underlying principle behind this model is working with clients' emotions. According to this model, behaviours are driven by emotion, which means that action is motivated by the emotional commitment that people have to achieve a given goal.

SUBJECT

What does your client want to talk about? What is his understanding of his goals?

TARGET IDENTIFICATION

It's pretty hard to hit a target that you can't see. Many people don't know exactly what they want, and, not knowing, don't know where to start. Not only must clients select a target, they also have to keep it in sight in order to hit it.

EMOTION

Emotions drive behaviour and that's why it's important for your client to have knowledge of how her emotions could be affecting her motivation towards achieving a goal. Is the goal worth it? If she can't answer that question, then spend some time searching for goals that do, or learning ways to overcome her aversions.

PERCEPTION AND CHOICE

You can understand your clients' particular perception. By consciously engaging in asking what something 'means' to them, coaches can help clients choose the route they want to take towards achieving a goal.

PLAN

Every plan is actually a process. You constantly have to revise, look at and course correct. While the shortest way to two points is a straight line, we all know that life is complicated and we should remain flexible enough to change course if needed.

PACE

Pay attention next time you're driving on the road, and you'll notice distance markers every so often; these are meant to give you an idea of how far you've gone. When establishing goals, you and your clients need to know and have a system to measure their progress. When will they achieve their goals?

ADAPT OR ACT

Every coaching model is intended to move clients into action, that is their commitment to themselves. It takes time, and sooner or later they'll realize that by taking that first step and then another, and another, and another, they'll eventually reach their destination.

The WHAT coaching model

This is more of a strategy than a model, one that you can use to discover what is behind behaviours. When someone asks us why we did something, we want to be consistent with what we say and the question why, tends to make us feel as if we need to justify ourselves, as if we're being judged. What ends up happening is that we tend to cling to our views and blocking our ability to see other perspectives.Something similar happens when we're asked the question how. On simple problems this question may be easily answered, but rarely is a problem simple and answering this question is likely to involve having to come up with different processes, all of which requires a lot of effort.

WHAT is the better question:

- If you can get this, just the way you want it, WHAT is the best thing about it?

- Okay, so WHAT is the first step to take to have that?

- WHAT will you do by next week?

- WHAT is the main obstacle that's preventing you from getting this?

- WHAT would it take to get past this block?

- If you could freely overcome these obstacles, WHAT would that mean for you?

- WHAT is the main thing you got out of this session?

When you ask what, your client is focusing her mind on a single item, one that's not looking for a reason or is too difficult to answer. It very often provides us with a simple way to find a solution, regardless of what she's answering.

Motivational interviewing

Motivational interviewing (MI) came about as a therapeutic counselling approach for treating alcohol abuse and was first described by W.R. Miller (1983). In context, as a model for eliciting change, it is useful as a coaching approach and needs to be in your coaching toolbox.

MI helps clients explore and resolve ambivalence and find the best possible solution. Like coaching, it's goal driven and focused towards solving internal conflict and bring about change. MI is non-judgemental, non-confrontational and non-adversarial. Change is sought from the client and is not imposed by a coach from the outside. It helps by identifying clients' intrinsic values and goals with the goal of stimulating intrinsic behavioural change. A coach will guide clients to express the ambivalence and work towards an acceptable outcome in line with their values. MI pursues this goal by asking questions and acting as a soundboard for clients to resolve their own conflict and bring about change. Coaches help by being the catalyst through which clients can envisage a better future and become increasingly motivated to achieve it. It allows people to think differently about their behaviour and ultimately to consider what might be gained by changing. MI is shaped by a guiding philosophy and understanding of what triggers change. Its guiding principles are:

- expressing empathy; coaches share their understanding of the clients' perspective with clients

- developing discrepancy, which help clients appreciate the value of change by exploring the discrepancy between how they want their lives to be vs. how they currently are (or the difference between their deeply held values and their day-to-day behaviour)

- rolling with resistance; clients accept reluctance to change as natural rather than pathological

- supporting self-efficacy; clients explicitly embrace autonomy (even when clients choose to not change) and move towards change successfully and with confidence.

Inside tip

I'd like to introduce you to my coaching model, the HEALTH Coaching Model:

HARMONY	Creating harmony through integration
EMPOWER	Empowering through self-responsibility
ATTTITUDE	Creating an open attitude
LINK	Making links in our life between mind and body
TRANSCEND	Transcending limiting mindsets
HEAL	Healing on all levels

Further coaching models

Paradigm coaching: Exploring the current set of beliefs and values in relation to realities and making adjustments for change.

Solution coaching: Recognizing issues and their source before moving on to solutions.

Zen coaching: Surrendering to what is happening and finding balance through acceptance.

Leap coaching: Challenging clients to something that is bigger than their comfort zone.

Strategic coaching: Identification of opportunity and deciding the role you will play before creating and monitoring a plan.

Performance coaching: Developing a compelling goal and creating milestones to keep the client goal focused.

Turnaround coaching: The deliberate identification of problems to determine cause and effect and then to restore integrity through the establishment of new goals.

Personal foundation model: Works on boundaries and standards. The higher clients want to go, the deeper their foundations must be.

Extreme self-care coaching: The redesigning and simplifying of one's life.

Grace coaching: Teaching clients to have faith in themselves, be generous to others and finding the joy in accomplishing meaningful things.

Paradox coaching: The recognition of conflict and understanding of both sides, without trying to resolve them and to find balance within the paradox.

Shift coaching: Shifting perspective to inquire and move forward on a new track.

Recovery coaching: Used when recovering from addictions, perceived loss or failure. Instead of denial or resistance, accept and move on.

Deep coaching: Digging deep into clients' belief systems to bring to light faulty beliefs, which can then be aligned with today's reality.

Bigger thinking: Challenging assumptions and expanding thinking to break out of the comfort zone.

Vision coaching: Identify a trend, extrapolate it into the future (the vision) and to take advantage of that trend today.

Distinction coaching: Reorienting from an old way of doing something to a new way of doing something.

Quality of life coaching: Re-evaluating life values.

Acceptance coaching: Accepting a weakness and using it to advantage.

Traditional coaching: Empathizing and feeling what the client feels, acting as a confidant and guide.

Intermediate coaching: Client and coach collaborate on developing goals and on achieving them.

Personal evolution: Evolution helps clients become different people by changing their environments.

Innovation coaching: This model centres on innovation, experimentation and creativity.

Attraction coaching: As clients add value to their lives, they attract feedback and opportunities.

3-D coaching: This model works on who one is, what one wants and how to get it.

Linear coaching: How to set the goal, create the plan, take action and hold oneself accountable.

Advanced coaching: Good for making a meaningful break from the past, to engage with new things and new ways of doing them.

Integrity coaching: A diagnostic tool to separate wants and needs.

Block removal coaching: A method to unblock the flow of energy (caused by limited beliefs and faulty thinking) causing resistance to growth.

The importance of client motivation

In order to achieve anything, we need to be motivated. Motivation can be externally or internally driven. We can be motivated by reward or penalty. There is a difference between 'want' and 'need' motivation. A want motivation is driven by enjoyment and personal preferences. The trick to keeping a client motivated is to identify his 'want' motivations, such as changing jobs (the want is more money) or losing weight (the want is feeling more attractive).

Psychologist Abraham Maslow introduced his concept of a hierarchy of needs in his 1943 paper 'A theory of human motivation' and his subsequent book, *Motivation and Personality* (1954). This hierarchy of needs affects people's motivations and decisions:

Self-actualization: Desire to become whatever you are capable of becoming, creativity, determining your own life patterns.

Aesthetic needs: Symmetry, order and beauty.

Cognitive needs: To know, understand and explore.

Self-esteem: Status, recognition and respect.

Belonging and love needs: Love, acceptance, membership of groups.

Safety: Protection from danger.

Physiological: Food, water, shelter.

The more basic needs like those at the bottom need to be satisfied as a matter of survival. As we go up the hierarchy, we can see the needs become more subtle, and maybe more challenging.

As a wellness coach, you are in a position of motivating others. If your client is unmotivated, he won't be receptive to your motivational efforts and is likely to resent you for showing what he might see as a patronizing attitude. In order to solve the problem, you need to know the symptoms and origin of the problem: what shows a lack of motivation and why there is a lack of motivation. Once you have this information, you can then create ways to motivate your client and overcome behavioural issues. Behavioural indicators of a lack of motivation in your client include:

- showing lack of initiative in completing challenging tasks
- no desire to improve self
- little interest in achieving established goals
- clock-watching
- beginning to come late (or not at all!).

Working with procrastination

When your clients procrastinate, they are likely to lack motivation. Overcoming the procrastination, which presents as a lack of motivation, involves examining beliefs. Exploring how these beliefs and fears operate are important keys to improving and maintaining motivation.

One reason for procrastination is the belief that the action will have a negative consequence. The client may think she is going to fail or that something will go wrong. Consequently, the client will delay the behaviour to try to avoid the negative consequence. For example, a client may:

- put off not bringing work home as part of her work/life balance plan, because she is afraid of being made redundant
- put off losing weight because he is afraid of facing the emotions he covers when comfort eating
- put off being assertive with friends because he fears the friend will get angry and dump him.

Although irrational, these fears can impede the client's ability to act. You need to coach the client through how to think about what the underlying fears are about and to evaluate whether that fear is realistic. The client needs to reframe faulty thinking by shifting the focus from the outcome to the process, which means greater self-awareness as the procrastination process occurs. As the cognitive awareness increases and is reframed, the behaviour will improve. Procrastination will reduce and achievement can occur which will reinforce the positive. Of course, being realistic, not all outcomes are positive, but by identifying possible risks, failure is reduced and the positive is still reinforced.

Motivation will significantly increase as the client understands and overcomes the deeper procrastination reasons and learns to take action in spite of the fears. Let's look at some common fears behind procrastination:

FEAR OF BEING IMPERFECT

Perfectionism is related to the client's fear of failure and the belief that everything she does needs to be perfect. Perfectionism is setting oneself up with an impossible standard to meet. Rather than experiencing a failure to meet an unreasonable expectation, she may just put off taking any action. To overcome this belief, help her realize that it is impossible to do everything perfectly, and it is the mistakes and failures that help her to grow and develop. It is the process that is important, not the final outcome, so focus on helping her learn from errors and less-than-perfect results, and don't let expectations of perfection hold her back.

Inside tip

Other reasons for procrastination might include:

- Downright laziness. The client really can't be bothered. Someone else can wave a magic wand and if that doesn't work – do they care? Unlikely.
- They can't find enough time to do work towards their agreed goal. Maybe time management is needed before goals can be actively worked towards.

FEAR OF FAILURE

One of the strongest causes of procrastination is fear of failure. Because clients are unsure of succeeding in their action, they put it off in order to avoid the potential failure. If they never actually do it, there's no way to fail, but not taking action ensures a failure because they don't accomplish anything. Rather than seeing failure as a negative outcome, reframe the situation as a learning experience. If things don't turn out as the client expected, he has learned what doesn't work, and that knowledge will help him do better next time. It is impossible to master anything without running into some unexpected problems, and the more understanding the client gets, the faster he can move towards achievement.

Inside tip

Clients may be approval-conscious of others and of you, the wellness coach. They may be keen to change and work towards goals, but be unsure the results will be good enough. You need to be mindful of how you give approval to clients. They may complete a task not always because they want to but so that you, the perceived authority figure, will smile and approve of them.

FEAR OF SUCCESS

By succeeding in a goal, clients may feel that they are obligated to continue succeeding in the future. The pressure to continue to succeed may become overwhelming, increasing their feelings of responsibility and stress. It may seem easier to put it off in order to avoid the additional burdens they associate with success. The solution lies in learning to embrace the concept that as they succeed in life, responsibility may increase, expectations may increase, but so does their power and freedom. Encourage clients not to hold themselves to unreasonable standards, and don't expect perfection every time, but help them be willing to raise their standards as they gain success.

FEAR OF IMPACTING RELATIONSHIPS

Another of the causes of client procrastination is a fear of how success will affect their relationships with others. If they succeed in implementing self-care strategies for their health issue, for example, will that strain the relationships with their partners who thrive on caring for them? It may seem easier to procrastinate just to maintain the status quo with those around them. It might also be that they are trying to do something to please someone else. Encourage your clients not to make the mistake of holding themselves back because of how they think people might react. First, it is impossible to predict how people will react. They may be surprised by finding that people are supportive for their success. Second, if others do have issues with your clients' succeeding, they may want to re-evaluate the importance of the relationship. Encourage them to focus on finding and celebrating their success and not to let other people hold them back.

Inside tip

I have had clients come to me for wellness coaching because their nearest and dearest care about them and have suggested it. The client wants to please someone else, but hasn't engaged with the idea on an inner level at all. Consequently, negotiated tasks aren't completed and they don't turn up to sessions.

FEAR OF REJECTION

A fear of rejection is one of the most common causes of procrastination. Putting oneself in front of others invites criticism. The uncertainty of how other people will react to your client can stop her from taking action and is especially true if she doesn't have much confidence in herself. Reframing rejection as feedback will help her improve her behaviour, rather than taking it as a personal attack.

Inside tips

Tips for motivating your clients:

- Get to know your clients' motivations by asking them.
- Ask your clients the reasons why they want to achieve their particular goal. (Ask them to write this list down and to read it when motivation falters.)
- Help clients understand the goal, the reason for it and its value.
- Encourage your clients to surround themselves with optimistic people.
- Coach your clients in setting clear and realistic goals (and break them down into small steps).
- Involve your clients in the wellness coaching process; don't tell them what to do.
- Encourage your clients to trust their capabilities to achieve something.
- If your clients are usually motivated but seem to be flagging, maybe they need a break.
- Encourage your clients to understand that failures are learning experiences.

CHANGE ASSOCIATIONS TO BEHAVIOURS

This technique is not so much fear driven as about making links between mindset and behaviour. Another step in stopping procrastination is to change associations to behaviour. For example, when your client puts off doing a task because there is something much more enjoyable to do, he is reinforcing the habit of procrastination. He begins to associate procrastination with enjoyment. Coach him to stop rewarding (enjoyment) the bad habit (procrastination) and start to associate pain (delayed effects of procrastination) immediately with the act of procrastinating.

MOVE FROM SHORT-TERM TO LONG-TERM MINDSET

Fear is not the motivator for this mindset either. Ask your clients to consider what they will miss out over the long-term if they don't do the things they need to do or have agreed to do, and the stress of chewing over the guilt of procrastination. Considering only the short-term consequences encourages procrastination, but if they consider what the long-term consequences are, they will be more motivated to stop procrastination.

The importance of managing change

> The only people who like change are busy cashiers and wet babies.
>
> *(Anonymous)*

Most people perceive change as a threat and tend to respond with a fight-or-flight mindset. We all try to avoid change if we can. We cut ourselves off through passivity and ignore what is happening. Or we might fight and actively resist change through negativity.

There are changes which are hoisted upon your clients from outside, such as redundancy, and then there are the changes they choose, such as wanting to lose weight. Change management is linked to control and security issues.

Every change can bring an opportunity; therefore clients have the choice of seeing change as a means of achieving their goals or as a barrier preventing them from reaching them. Humans are wonderfully capable of adapting to a wide variety of environments and situations. Realizing this can help your clients to embrace and work with change rather than avoiding or fighting it. Change the mindset then the behaviour will change. If clients believe that there is nothing they can do to influence an outcome, nothing will change. But if they believe that they've got unlimited potential, anything can change.

Some of the things your client might seek to change include:

Stress	⟶ Relaxation
Physical illness	⟶ Realistic health
Imbalance	⟶ Balance
Powerlessness	⟶ Empowerment
Negative attitude	⟶ Positive outlook
Fragmentation of mind	⟶ Integration of mind
Being reactive	⟶ Being proactive

What you are helping clients to change is their mindset, which in turn will affect their behaviours and therefore their wellness.

Phases of change

When planning to manage change as part of wellness coaching, bear in mind that everyone reacts to change differently. To help you manage client change, understand the six major phases of change (which are similar to the grieving process):

STAGE 1: SHOCK AND DENIAL

Client mindset: Shock, disbelief, not feeling in control.

Client behaviour: Asking 'Why' instead of 'How', denial, resistance, not seeking support, paralysis, procrastinating.

STAGE 2: SEARCHING

Client mindset: Although wellness goals may have been identified at this stage, the client may be unsure of what to expect as a result of a possible change, so she anticipates what the future holds. Client expectations may or may not be realistic. She may feel overwhelmed, powerless or impatient for it to be alright.

Client behaviour: Asking 'why' instead of 'how', dwelling on what she doesn't like, procrastinating, a sense of 'hopping' from solution to solution.

STAGE 3: CONFRONTATION

Client mindset: Clients begin to confront the reality of possible change in relation to wellness. They might feel overwhelmed and powerless. They may experience this phase with impatience, excitement, anger or fear.

Client behaviour: Asking 'Why' instead of 'How', resistance, dwelling on what they don't like, procrastinating.

STAGE 4: REALIZATION

Client mindset: As the wellness change begins to bite, clients realize that nothing is ever going to be the same. They may feel impatient, powerless or overwhelmed.

Client behaviour: Dwelling on what they don't like, procrastinating, asking 'why' instead of 'how'.

STAGE 5: DEPRESSION

Client mindset: Change often involves a loss; for example, loss of perfect health or loss of a perceived pay-off. This loss necessitates a grieving process and fears which may need to be dealt with. This is the stage where clients mourn the past. Not only have they realized the change intellectually, but now they begin to comprehend it emotionally as well. They may not feel in control. They might feel overwhelmed.

Client behaviour: Dwelling on what they don't like, asking 'why' instead of 'how'.

STAGE 6: ACCEPTANCE

Client mindset: This is where clients begin to emotionally accept the wellness-related change. Although they might still be doubtful, they no longer fight the change. It is hoped that this is the beginning of positive acceptance and movement forward and not passive acceptance and apathy.

Client behaviour: Asking 'how' instead of 'why'.

Decision-making styles

Realizing what clients' normal decision-making style is can enable us to develop personal change-management tactics in relation to wellness. These four decision-making styles detailed in *Managing with Style: A Guide to Understanding, Assessing and Improving Decision-Making* (1987) by Alan J. Rowe and Richard O. Mason have the following characteristics:

- Analytical coping strategy: Clients see change as a challenging puzzle to be solved with time required to gather information and draw conclusions. Clients resist change if they are not given enough time to think it through.

- Conceptual coping strategy: Clients are interested in how change fits into the big picture. They want to be involved in defining what needs to change and why. Clients will resist change if they feel excluded from participating in the change process.

- Behavioural coping strategy: Clients want to know how everyone feels about the changes ahead. They work best when they know there is support for the change. If the change adversely affects someone close to them, they will perceive change as a crisis.

- Directive coping strategy: Clients want specifics on how the change will affect them and what their own role will be during the process. If they know the rules of the change process and the desired outcome, they will act rapidly to achieve change goals. They resist change if the rules or anticipated results are not clearly defined.

Here are three things to bear in mind with change management. First, not everyone will change at the same rate. Some of your clients may adapt rapidly while others take more time. Second, sometimes the results of change may come more slowly than your clients would like. Third, some clients may find the journey uncomfortable and force (unrealistic) change due to wanting it over as soon as possible.

Encourage your clients to view change as the 'new normalcy' of their wellness life. The sooner they can accept that these changes are permanent, the better they can cope with them and reap their benefits.

Inside tips

In 1999, I developed breast cancer. As I prepared for a mastectomy, I felt as if I were losing everything. I went through a massive change internally. To help myself through this time, I:

- looked for how could I take better care of myself
- asked myself if and how I wanted to redefine my life goals
- took pleasure in simple rituals such as watching *Coronation Street*, going for a daily walk around familiar landscapes, writing regularly in my journal
- took one day at a time
- kept positive; e.g. 'I will get through this'
- had realistic expectations, e.g. I may have to have radiotherapy or chemotherapy
- built a support network which offered a wide range of different options, such as someone to give hugs, someone to show me her mastectomy and reconstructed boob
- became informed so I could anticipate possible challenges.

Keeping a personal wellness journal

Journalling or personal writing takes many forms. Its history is rooted as far back as the tenth century in Japan, when pillow books were used to record daily lives and thoughts. Today, the term *journalling* is usually used for personal writing that explores the inner world of the self.

Clients can jot down their thoughts and feelings in their personal journal in between wellness coaching sessions. Journalling can:

- help clients know themselves better through clarifying thoughts and feelings

- reduce stress, as writing about painful emotions helps to release the intensity of these feelings

- solve problems more effectively (we problem solve from a left-brained, analytical perspective but often the answer can only be found by engaging right-brained creativity and intuition – writing unlocks these other capabilities to release creative solutions)

- work through issues that wellness coaching has uncovered

- allow clients to track patterns and improvement over time.

R. Bruce (1998) describes research with subjects who journal led about traumatic experiences and most of them generally experienced improved physical health. Adams (1998) also talks about journalling as therapy for enhancing psychological healing and growth.

Journalling techniques

Here are six techniques you can use with your wellness coaching clients:

REFLECTIVE WRITING

Ask your clients to write about events that are happening to them or around them, such as life changes or illness. Start with 'It was a time when___' then describe the event in detail, encouraging clients to use as many senses as possible. What were the sounds, smells, sights, feelings, etc. that were present? Tell the client to write about the event as though he were observing himself. Tell the client to use 'she' and 'he' rather than 'I' in his sentences and describe the activities as an outside observer, as this helps give perspective to an otherwise very personal experience.

MAKE A LIST

Some ideas for your clients: 25 ways they could nurture themselves, 15 things they could do to improve their lives, 10 nourishing treats.

CATHARTIC WRITING

Ask your clients to write about their feelings. Put their pain, fear, anger, frustrations, and grief down on paper. The journal won't judge or criticize them. They can use it as a safe place to let out everything they feel. Sometimes they may choose to throw away their writing or burn it as a ritual way of letting it go. Clients can begin with the phrase, 'Right now I feel___' then let themselves write whatever comes out. If they run out of feelings, ask them to re-read what they've just written and then write the next thing that comes to mind.

FOOD JOURNAL

If your client is on a diet or looking for food intolerance, ask her to detail all she eats and drinks in a journal. She can add her reasons for eating and her feelings at the time she ate/drank. She might see some patterns she can break.

UNSENT LETTERS

Your clients can write a letter in their journals to a person, place, event or belief. The journal gives them a powerful way to express what they experience and feel about any situation, when they may not feel comfortable doing it more directly. This technique is especially helpful in dealing with death, endings or separation. Begin with a salutation, just as they would if they were writing a letter: 'Dear___.'

DIALOGUE
Ira Progoff, the grandfather of personal journal writing and author of *At a Journal Workshop* (1992), has developed a full list of dialogues your client may want to use. A client could dialogue with:

- a person, present or past relationships, living or deceased
- events, situations, decisions and circumstances
- an enigmatic dream or a symbol, person or situation in a dream that you want to know more about
- a particular emotion you might want to have a conversation with.

Supporting your client

Your client could do some journalling during a session or in between sessions. It is the client's choice whether to show you the work, read it to you or just share the gist of it. Don't forget the journal. It is a client tool, but the results from it can be used in the coaching sessions.

Inside tips

- You could offer group coaching or workshops on using journalling for wellness
- Use journalling as part of your remote coaching wellness coaching programme

---

Wellness coaching networks

Networking is a two-way process to make contacts for professional support for your wellness coaching business and your clients. Networking with different clusters will help:

- raise your profile
- build a client referral network
- generate sales
- open up diversification opportunities

- expand your knowledge
- support your development.

Client-related networks
Wellness networks can be client related, for example: on- and offline course providers, support personnel for cultural/ethnic issues, bodywork therapists, counsellors and psychotherapists, mindbody therapists, mental health agencies, bereavement agencies, benefit support, local council agencies, helplines, local support groups, CABs, condition-led organizations like Cancerbackup, and career-management specialists.

CPD-related networks
Network with the professional associations you belong to, keep an eye on therapy or coaching-specific courses which will increase your knowledge and skills base and don't forget courses which build your business skills! You also need your network of coaches, supervisors and mentors for support and development.

Social networking
Social networking is a means of communicating and sharing information on an online community. Through these virtual communities you can access associates, developing a platform to generate leads and establish yourself as a recognized expert.

Define what you have to give and what benefits you expect to receive from connecting with people online. Whom do you want to connect with? What industries? With what objectives? What do you have to offer? Use these platforms to build contacts, for business development objectives and to offer your expertise.

Your best route for finding niche communities is connecting with some of the people in that target group via the larger, public networks. Get to know them and find out where else they connect. Many niche communities will not be highly visible as networking sites. They may just be email discussion lists and hard to discover through search engines.

Some of the best sites for business development purposes are: BizNik, XING, NFP, Facebook, ZoomInfo, FastPitchNetworking, LinkedIn, Twitter, Ziggs, Ryze, Bebo, BizWiz and Ecademy.

In addition, you could use bulletin boards (web pages where you can view and post questions/comments on a specific subject). Discussion lists are similar to bulletin boards but are emailed to members of the list. You could network through live chats. If you subscribe to an online service offering interactive channels like MSN or CompuServe, entire areas may be dedicated to your profession or target market.

Much of the benefit of online networking is in building your business passively by creating an attractive profile for yourself. Create a profile that gives people enough information about both you and your business to determine if you might be a good connection. Include details about your recent professional history and interests, and any personal interests which you are willing to make public and use as a basis for connecting.

These online communities don't work unless you work them. You can't expect to derive value from your participation unless you are also willing to create value. Watch for opportunities to contribute your expertise to the public conversation, or to make connections between others, just as you would want others to do for you.

Strategic business networking

This networking route is about partnerships. There is a sense of coming together, exploring how the relationship may be mutually beneficial and working together to make it so. This makes strategic business networking much safer in a business social situation than selling or marketing. Suggestions of possible partnerships don't set off the automatic defence mechanisms when we are being sold or marketed to. It's always easier to talk about a partnership than a purchase.

Inside tip

Hold volunteer positions in organizations. This is a great way to put back into the community and stay visible as a wellness expert.

CPD task sheet

This is your Continuing Professional Development (CPD) task sheet which summarizes key module points and offers you the opportunity to engage with tasks to deepen your learning.

Module summary

- There are differences between coaching, counselling and mentoring and an occassional overlap is possible within the wellness coaching model.
- Lifecycles produce changing wellness needs.
- How people learn influences how they engage with the wellness coaching process.
- There are a variety of coaching models to use.
- Client motivation is key to the success of wellness coaching.
- Change management is an important area for coaching clients.
- Wellness journalling can be a profound inclusion within wellness coaching.
- Networking for both client support and professional development is crucial.

Your tasks

1. Reflect on how lifecycle changes your clients' wellness needs.
2. Reflect on your past and present clients and their different lifecycles and wellness needs.
3. How do you like to learn?
4. Use different coaching models on friends and colleagues.
5. What is your motivation for incorporating wellness coaching into your practice?
6. Consider the last major change in your life and how you managed it.
7. What are your networks for client support and professional development?

Wellness Coaching Skills Toolkit

Part 2 offers a practical toolkit of wellness coaching skills you can begin to integrate into your therapeutic practice.

Module 4: Core Skills Set

Module 5: Cognitive Behavioural Coaching

Module 6: Additional Skills for Wellness Coaching

Module 4
Core Skills Set

By the end of this module, you will understand:

- How to use the Wellness Coaching Intro-Pack
- How to use body language
- How to use powerful questioning
- How to use active listening
- How to develop client rapport
- How to provide constructive feedback
- How to facilitate the opening wellness coaching session
- How to facilitate ongoing wellness coaching sessions
- How to coach a skill
- How to end the wellness coaching relationship

Wellness Coaching Intro-Pack

Having set the scene for wellness coaching, we're now ready to move into the nitty gritty of delivery.

The Wellness Coaching Intro-Pack (Form 4.1) is designed to be emailed or given to the client prior to the first wellness coaching session. It provides information which can be used in the first session and as a basis to the Personal Wellness Plan (PWP, Form 4.3). Feel free to change it to suit.

There is also an example Wellness Coaching Agreement (Form 4.2) for the client to sign at the first meeting.

All the forms in this module that are designed to be filled in by clients are available at www.jkp.com/catalogue/book/9781848190634/resources.

Inside tip

The Wellness Coaching Intro-Pack isn't compulsory. The information gleaned from the pack is useful as a blueprint in order to get to know your client and her initial goals. It is also useful for the client to reflect on. If you don't want to use this plan or something like it, you will need to talk through with the client, her perceived goals. It might be that you're eager to use the Wellness Coaching Intro-Pack, but your client is unwilling to complete it.

Based on this information, you can co-create the wellness coaching plan. Remember that this information is to be used in an organic way. As your client moves through the wellness coaching process, her aims and objectives will organically change.

At the start of the wellness coaching process, your client's goals may be unrealistic and somewhat large, so you will need to go through several processes to help her focus on the real issues.

Form 4.1
Wellness Coaching Intro-Pack

As your wellness coach, it is important that I understand how you view yourself and your life. Complete the questions as fully as you can and either email them to me in advance of our first session or bring them with you.

Name: Email:

GP:

Land-line: Mobile:

Age: Occupation:

Address:

Coaching
What has influenced your decision to work with a wellness coach at this time?

What do you want from the wellness coaching relationship?

What is the best way for me to coach you most effectively?

Physical wellness
Detail past illnesses:

Detail past hospitalization/surgery:

Detail your diet (give an example of a typical day's eating/drinking):

Detail any supplements (vitamins, minerals) or herbs you're taking:

Detail your activity/exercise level:

Describe any health challenges that you currently experience (major concerns in addition to problems like headaches, insomnia, etc.):

Detail any medication and the intended impact of the medication:

Psychological wellness
Detail any mental health issues you have had in the past or currently have:

What do you do to reduce stress in your life?

Social wellness
Who is the one special person you could contact if you needed help?

In general, how many relatives, other than your children, do you feel close to and have contact with at least once a month?

In general, how many friends do you feel close to and have contact with at least once a month?

Whom can you count on for emotional support (talking over problems or helping you make a decision)?

To what extent do you participate in community activities?

 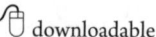 downloadable

Occupational wellness
Detail your current paid work status:

Detail your current community or volunteer work status:

What do you do that is meaningful to you to occupy your time?

How do your occupational (paid or unpaid) goals support your personal goals or sense of purpose?

Environmental wellness
In what ways are you proactive in practising environmental management (animals, land, resources) within your community?

How do you practise good ergonomics within your workplace?

Spiritual wellness
What is your spiritual base or belief system?

How do you draw upon your spiritual beliefs for support and help in moving forward with your life?

Please describe what gives you a sense of purpose in life. What activities have meaning or heart for you?

What's missing in your life, the presence of which would make your life more fulfilling?

Focusing your choices

This exercise will add clarity to the primary areas you want to focus on in wellness coaching. Please describe the five lifestyle areas you would like to change or improve. How will it look when you accomplish your goals?

1. I would like to improve or change…

    How will your wellness change when this is improved or changed?

2. I would like to improve or change…

    How will your wellness change when this is improved or changed?

3. I would like to improve or change…

    How will your wellness change when this is improved or changed?

4. I would like to improve or change…

    How will your wellness change when this is improved or changed?

5. I would like to improve or change…

    How will your wellness change when this is improved or changed?

Form 4.2
Wellness Coaching Agreement

As a wellness coaching client, I:

- am fully responsible for my choices and decisions during my wellness coaching sessions

- am aware that I can choose to discontinue wellness coaching at any time

- understand that wellness coaching does not treat mental health issues and is not a substitute for medical treatment, and that professional referrals will be given if needed

- understand that wellness coaching can facilitate the development and implementation of my wellness goals across different areas of my life

- promise that if I am under the care of a mental health professional, I have discussed with them the possibility of working with a wellness coach and that agreement has been reached that I may do so

- understand that information will be held confidential unless I state otherwise in writing, except as required by law or in supervision

- understand that wellness coaching is not to be used in lieu of medical treatment or professional guidance in other life areas, and that I will seek appropriate advice when required.

Client: _____ Date:_____

How to use body language

Body language is the art of non-verbal communication. Mindfulness of our own body language as well as observing that of our client is vital when coaching. We need to demonstrate positive body language in order to build rapport. Clients may not be aware of their body language and may show mixed messages via what they say and how their body presents, which can be revealing and helpful to the coaching process.

The four elements of body language

The four elements of body language are:

FACE

Your face is a major source of expression when communicating with others, for example the colour of skin, mouth position, what you do with your nose and the eyes.

The colour of the skin can redden, for example through blushing (embarrassment or intense emotion) or through anger. The face can whiten with anger or shock.

If we look at the mouth position, it might be that the client is chewing her lip (anxiety) or pursing it through annoyance (what I call the 'cat's bum' look). Sometimes the pursing of the lips is the client trying not to say something she wants to. A hand in front of the mouth is a blocking behaviour. It also makes it hard to read the client if you can't see her mouth when she is talking. Some clients smile their way through an entire session no matter how stressed or angry they are (the 'people pleaser' grin). Sometimes this inane grin seems like a clown's mask to cover inner distress. The mouth can go into a thoughtful grimace, indicating the client is working something through. Then there's the fearful lip-licking behaviour.

Let's move onto the nose. I'm a nose-twitcher myself (which also involves moving the mouth – so look for the two together). My students recognize if I do this, I'm doubting something. Touching the nose might indicate a lie – touching the nose tends to partially cover the mouth, so look beneath the surface of what your client is saying.

Finally, the eyes have it. When we look at someone, we tend to go in a T-shape, across from one eye to the other and then down to the mouth. (As an aside, the lower down the body we go, the more intimate we are, or want to be, with the other person!) Direct eye contact with occasional blinking is positive. If clients look to the left or right of you or above you or consistently out of the window, I would suggest they are avoiding eye contact. What else are they avoiding? It is natural when we are thinking deeply to move our eyes away from another. We think, regroup and then resume eye contact again. That's fine. Eye blinking shows brain activity, too much blinking might be distress or reduced eye blinking might indicates a switching off (I can always tell when my husband has had a bit to drink because his blinking rate goes down to about once a minute – or less!). Direct gazing at you without blinking at all might indicate some kind of psychological shut-down in process, that the client doesn't understand something, or it might be that she's tired or under the weather. Then you've got the eye-shutting, which is a kind of withdrawal or very deep thinking. If you notice eye activity that you're not sure of, ask the client what is happening for her at that moment. Learn to read the eyes. It is possible to see a range of emotions and thoughts through the eyes that the lips may not say.

VOICE

Your voice is not only used to verbalize language, it is an integral part of your non-verbal communication. Your tone of voice, volume, emotion and pace influence the messages you send as part of your body language.

If your clients are unsure, they may mumble, squeak or speak fast. When angry, their voice might rise (they might also be fearful) and have a speedy pace. A voice may sound controlled but be loaded with intensity. Be mindful also that medication, alcohol or drugs might influence how someone sounds.

Inside tip

As a wellness coach, you need to communicate effectively during your sessions and to use language that has the greatest positive impact on the client. You will elicit a better response from your client if your communication is clear and articulate. Use language that is appropriate and respectful to the client, for example non-sexist, non-racist, non-technical and non-jargon.

Also use the language the client uses; for example if they use casual language, you use it. The effect of language is interesting. I remember once – and this isn't something I suggest you do ad hoc – at a business meeting for a training contract to work with youngsters, I swore (mildly!). At the end of the meeting, I was offered the contract. I asked why I was offered the work. The boss said among other reasons, it was because I swore. It showed I was human and I would speak the youngster's language just fine.

GESTURES

Your gestures can be related or unrelated to verbal communication. For example, as part of saying hello, you might wave at another person but not actually say the word out loud. Or, you might use hand gestures to emphasize a key point during a presentation in which case, your gesture is related to the verbal communication. Some people are more hand flappers than others, either by inclination or culture. Clients will sometimes use their hands to emphasize a point, like pushing away something or someone.

POSTURE

Your posture includes how you tilt your head, slump your shoulders and how you position legs, arms, and hips. Each of these parts of your body work separately as well as together to send non-verbal cues.

If clients are feeling motivated, their posture will be upright and open with direct eye contact. If they are feeling distressed, they might be slumped. An unwillingness to engage tends to be shown with crossed arms and legs or a turning of the body away from the speaker. Crossed arms with an unblinking stare is more hostile. Hands up behind the head, often adapted by men, is a desire to feel more in control (you could be getting under the skin, if your client does this one).

Inside tip

You will be using positive body language awareness in relation to how you present yourself to your clients. You will also be using body language to read your clients and how they match what they are saying with how their body speaks. Does what they say match what you see?

The mirroring technique

Mirror the physiology of your clients. If they are down, go down to their level. If they are up, come up to their level. If they are talking fast, you talk fast. If they are slouching, you slouch. Then, as you are talking with them, slowly begin to make small changes in your body. Your goal is to bring the person you are trying to influence into the physiology that will be most effective for getting your end outcome.

Emotional shifts

Non-verbal cues will help you identify when the client has experienced an emotional shift. Watch for changes in facial expression, shift in posture or body position and tightening of muscles. Verbal cues might include a change in voice tone, pitch, volume or pace. Other signs might include mumbling or sighs. Having noticed a change, you can ask, 'What was going through your mind just now?' or 'What's happening for you?'

How to use powerful questioning

A key skill of the wellness coach is the ability to ask questions which reveal the information needed for clarification of the client's issues. It also focuses your thoughts and actions when responding. There are basically two types of questions, open and closed.

Open questions widen out the dialogue because the client has to give a considered answer. In order to work with a client, we need to know more of what the client is feeling and thinking, wanting and planning. But our usual yes/no questions tend to shut people up rather than opening them up. Open-ended questions allow for a wide range of responses. For example, asking, 'What did you think of autogenic training?' will evoke a more detailed response than 'Did you like autogenic training?' which could be answered with a yes or no. One of our goals is to facilitate change. We can't do a good job of that unless we address the client's concerns. We won't understand those concerns unless we ask questions that invite discussion.

Closed questions restrict the response of the other person to a yes or a no answer. For example, 'Did you think the visualization exercise was useful?' is closed, while 'What did you think of the visualization exercise?' is open and widens the response out. Here are some examples of open-ended questions.

Personal responsibility questions

These imply that others have the responsibility for owning a problem and making choices that contribute to solving it. For example:

- What skills might you develop in order to help you with this problem?
- Where do you feel stuck?
- How are you managing the situation?
- What can you do to help yourself?
- What are your priorities at the moment?
- Why do you think that is?
- How do you think you can contribute to (easing the situation)?
- Why do you think that?
- What could you do to change?
- How might you achieve_____?

- What's your role in this issue?
- What can you do for yourself?
- What's preventing you from_____?
- What would you be willing to give up for that?
- If you could change one thing, what would it be?
- Imagine a point in the future where your issue is resolved. How did you get there?

Feeling questions

These questions elicit feelings generated by a problem. For example:

- How do you feel about that?
- In what other ways is the situation affecting you?
- How are you feeling at the moment?
- If I could get inside your head, what would this (anger) look like?
- How do you feel about what we've discussed?

Specification questions

These types of questions focus in on the details of the problem. For example:

- When you say 'he keeps badgering you', what exactly do you mean?
- Where do you feel stuck?
- What is the intent of what you're saying?
- In what other ways is the situation affecting you?
- Can you explain how your (anger) comes out?
- How are you feeling at the moment?
- What do you think the problem is?
- If I could get inside your head, what would this (anger) look like?
- What's stopping you from moving forward on this?

Elaboration questions

Ones that give others the chance to expand what they're talking about. For example:

- What else would you like to tell me?
- Where do you feel stuck?

- What can I do for you?
- What do you think the problem is?
- What do you hope to get from these sessions?
- In what other ways is the situation affecting you?
- Is there anything you want to share in this session about_____?
- What has changed since we last met?
- What would help you move in the right direction?
- What, in the past, has helped you to (relax)?
- What's stopping you from moving forward on this?
- What is on your mind?
- Which areas do you feel you'd like to work on today?
- Is there anything else you'd like to tell me?
- Would you like to tell me more about_____?
- Why do you think that?
- What do you feel you've gained from this session?
- How do you feel about what we've discussed?
- Is there anything else you'd like to bring up in this session?
- What could you do to change?
- How might you achieve_____?

Inside tip

Ask *one* question at a time and give the client time to reflect and respond. Don't jump in with another question if the client is trying to process and there is a long silence.

How to use active listening

Poor listening equates to misunderstandings and time wasted between you and your client. It leads to lower productivity and lower morale. Most of us think we are good listeners. We spend up to 80 per cent of our waking hours either listening or acting on what we hear. Untrained listeners lose 75 per cent of what they hear in a matter of hours and often capture less than half of the message at the time they receive it (Lindahl 2009).

Active listening focuses completely on what the client is saying and not saying. The skill involves understanding the meaning of what is said in the context of the client's desires and to support the client's self-expression.

Do you hear or do you listen? What is the difference? We can all hear unless we have an impairment of some sort, but listening is more sophisticated. You could hear the client say, 'I'm happy with the changes I've made'. But if you listened to his tone of voice, how he said the words and his body language, you might pick up that he is confused and isn't feeling too confident about the changes. So instead of mindlessly accepting his words, you might consider asking what the problem is or how you could help him.

Inside tip

Hearing is one-dimensional. Listening is a multi-faceted activity.

Paraphrasing

In order to show active listening the wellness coach will use paraphrasing, which means summarizing in a few words what the client is saying. This is done in order to clarify your understanding of what is being said. Often we listen and assume we have understood another's meaning, when in reality we've got the wrong end of the stick. Paraphrasing can be periodically done throughout the conversation with your client to ensure you're on the right track of understanding. When you're on the right track, you're better placed to facilitate sessions. If you're on the wrong track, time is wasted in misunderstanding and avoidance of the real issues.

Depending upon the circumstances, it may be best to use the client's own words or use your own words. It is a matter of judgement to know how best to paraphrase, depending upon the situation. In order to paraphrase effectively we need a reasonable vocabulary, especially when it comes to putting feelings into words. For example:

Client: 'I feel under pressure with my children, and I don't always get my homework done, which I then feel bad about.'

Wellness coach: 'You feel concerned if you don't put your children first and this causes you to put your coursework on the back burner, which leads to more anxiety.'

Reflecting feelings

Reflecting feeling is similar to paraphrasing and is another useful skill within the coaching relationship. Your client may send voice and body messages that negate verbal messages. Bruce mutters, 'I'm OK' yet has angry eyes. A good reflection of feelings entails responding to a client's spoken and unspoken messages. Reflecting feelings involves sensing a client's flow of emotions and experiencing and communicating this back. For example:

> *Bruce to wellness coach:* 'I feel frustrated that I'm finding it so hard to stop smoking, especially after I've eaten. I get really ratty after my supper – that's my weakest time.'

> *Bruce's feelings words and phrases:* frustration, ratty

> *Reflection of feeling:* 'You feel frustrated and irritable when you want a cigarette, especially after your evening meal.'

Interferences to active listening

There can be many sources of interference in your listener such as:

hearing difficulties	sight difficulties
physical distractions	fatigue or illness
low attention span	time pressure
doubt about the trustworthiness of the coach	daydreaming
perceived lack of relevance	memory difficulties
limited vocabulary	sensitive topic area
feeling threatened	anger/other extreme emotions
personal need results in selective listening	not feeling accepted by coach
anxiety about what is required of them	they can't wait to say something

Your client might find it difficult to listen to you when you ramble and go off the subject, speak for too long, make too many points, become dogmatic or aren't sure of what you are trying to say.

Active listening means you have to attend to all the signals given off by the client – not only the sounds, but also using your sight to pick up the non-verbal signals. The purpose of this active listening is to pay attention to and try to understand the thoughts, feelings and behaviour of the client.

Inside tips

Ten skills of active listening:

- possessing an attitude of respect and acceptance
- tuning into the client's internal viewpoint
- sending good voice messages
- sending good body messages
- using openers, e.g. 'How have you been getting on?'
- paraphrasing
- reflecting feelings
- showing understanding of context and difference
- managing initial resistances
- using small rewards, e.g. brief expressions of interest such as, 'Yes, tell me more'.

How to develop client rapport

Creating a strong foundation of trust is how you develop rapport in your wellness coaching relationship. Coaching happens in a collaborative relationship based on mutual trust with a high degree of openness between both parties. Building trust should be a conscious effort for you, because coach–client relationships can sometimes begin with disempowering expectations that can cause clients to distrust their coach and withhold information. For example, a client may assume, based on her past experience of authority figures, that you are looking for ways to judge and criticize her.

As a wellness coach, you need to develop the ability to create a safe, supportive environment with your client that produces ongoing mutual respect and trust.

You always need to show genuine concern for the client's welfare and future and continuously demonstrate personal integrity, reliability, honesty and consistency. It is important to demonstrate respect for the client's perceptions, learning style and personal being.

Trust develops when you allow clients to vent the situation without judgement in order to move on to the next step, and rapport evolves as you hear your clients' concerns about what is and is not possible from their perspective. Give them a chance to be heard and listen beyond their words for deeper understanding of their intentions and needs. You can do this by encouraging and integrating the clients' expression of feelings, perceptions, concerns, beliefs and suggestions. You provide ongoing support for and champion new behaviours and actions, including those involving risk taking and fear of failure. Openly appreciate your clients and be generous with your praise, pointing out the specifics of their personality and behaviour that add value.

Inside tips

- Linking comments are words you might say to move from one section of dialogue to another. For example: 'Let's talk about this', 'Tell me more', 'The message I'm getting is__', 'I'm getting a sense of__', 'Take me back to a time when you felt__'.
- Provide the client with a sense of security and privacy during a session.
- Use your client's name.
- Ensure that noise does not affect communication.
- Create an ambient and neutral environment through décor, light and other facilities such as water on hand.
- Affirm the client's self-help strategies and achievements. Give the client plenty of positive strokes.
- Always acknowledge the client's emotional states.
- Encourage the client to utilize support outside of the wellness coaching sessions.
- Deal with the immediacy of what the client is saying or feeling.

Ask a lot of open-ended questions. People trust people who are interested in them. As a wellness coach, the more you use questioning to build rapport the more likely it is that your client will trust you and be coachable. When you ask a question, pause long enough to let the client answer. To build trust you must patiently provide an empty space for the answer to evolve from the client.

Consider Neil Fleming's VARK model as a way of identifying a client's preferred mode of communication in order to build rapport (see Module 3). Here is a list of phrases to help you identify a dominant mode:

- Visual language: It looks like___, in my mind's eye___, it's crystal clear, it's seems hazy, I take a dim view, I need to be up front, it appears to me___, you get the picture, it's clear cut, here's a bird's eye view.

- Kinesthetic language: I need to touch base with___, I'm conscious of___, you can sense___, you need to experience it, she perceived___, lay your cards on the table, I need to come to grips with it, I could pull some strings, I could hang on in there, it all boils down to___, we could start from scratch, hold on, that's a pain in the neck.

- Auditory language: I gave her an earful, it rings a bell, I'm all ears, I need to make myself heard, I'm tuned in, that's unheard of, to tell the truth___, listen up, I was tongue-tied, let me describe it, it sounds like___, just say it, in a manner of speaking___.

If your objective is to bring people to a new awareness, you must lead by helping them to feel comfortable. You can do this by mirroring their body language. It will help to build rapport, increase your clients' feelings of safety and their receptiveness to the coaching process. Mirroring creates a harmonious climate for your ideas because you are accepting the other person. Your acceptance leads to their acceptance of you. This enables you to successfully lead them into new areas of experience.

When coaching, behave as if your clients are your whole world. They are your world for that one or two hours you are with them. Focusing intently on them will build rapport. It will make them feel important and make it easier for them to trust you. If any issues arise for you, personal or professional, park them in your mind, refocus on your clients, and deal with the parked issues later in private or in supervision.

We all like to be cared about – it makes us feel good. If your client seems disappointed or down, ask, 'You seem down today; what is happening for you?' You needn't dwell on the concern, but showing you notice builds rapport and it might make the client's mind clear and ready for coaching. Make sure to bring the conversation back to its original intent with tact. Let your clients know you are pleased to see them and enjoy working with them.

One other way to build rapport is let your clients know that you understand where they are coming from. This creates rapport because people want to know that they have been heard. That makes them feel important and makes it easier for them to trust you. Being heard is a building block of trust. It's all about being an active listener. Remember: you don't have to agree, as long as you understand.

Building rapport is similar to strengthening a bridge over a river. The stronger the bridge and the clearer the way, the more it can carry – meaning the better rapport you have in a relationship with someone, the more you can ask of him, and the more effective the wellness coaching will be.

How to provide constructive feedback

Your clients need feedback. They need to know your response to what is happening to them, what their own thoughts and feelings are and how they might change and move on. Wellness coaching is a challenging environment for those coming to you. They may ask themselves questions such as:

- Can I change?
- What if I get it wrong?
- Where am I going with this?
- How can I fit these challenges in the rest of my life?
- What if I don't like the wellness coach?
- How can I understand this?
- Am I doing this right?
- Am I good enough?

Your feedback provides a sounding board to their questions. How you respond to their problems and solutions needs to give them confidence, insight and the motivation to move on.

Here are a few pointers for giving feedback. Acknowledge the positive achievements of the client. If the performance hasn't gone too well, empathize with the client's situation or feelings. When giving feedback, use the sandwich technique: give a positive, followed up with the constructive criticism or feedback and finish with a positive. For example, 'Looking at what you've done over the last week! You have put a lot of work in and that is a credit to you. However, it might be helpful if you focused on what you have achieved instead of looking at what you haven't. We are working together for another couple of months, and I'm sure with some time management, you can achieve what you want to.' Focus on client behaviour and let the feedback be well timed and as near the event as possible. See Table 4.1 for more ideas.

Table 4.1 Guidelines for giving feedback

Feedback is most useful when it is:	Feedback is least useful when it is:
specific	vague
focused on behaviour	impossible to change the situation
positive	negative
supportive	offering little or no support
given privately	given in front of others
based on first-hand information	hearsay and speculative
based on behaviour	a personality attack
uncluttered by evaluative judgements	judgemental
given with care	given thoughtlessly
easily acted on	hard to act upon
expressed directly	expressed indirectly or to someone else
well timed	delayed

Inside tip

It is useful to periodically ask your clients how they are with the process and outcomes of the wellness coaching sessions and with your performance. This is part of the co-creative process and places the ownership in your clients' hands. They have the right to give you feedback on how they are experiencing the sessions and how satisfied they are with the outcomes as well as how you are coaching them. You can agree, disagree or agree in part with what the clients present. Be adult (no matter how boosted up or crushed you may feel) and always respond positively.

How to facilitate the opening wellness coaching session

Prior to the first wellness coaching session, your clients will have completed the Wellness Coaching Intro-Pack. They will have emailed it to you or they might bring it with them. I don't want to be prescriptive in how you deliver the first session, but these steps may help clarify your thoughts and actions.

You will need to have identified whether your client wants face-to-face sessions or remote coaching.

Step 1: Clarify client expectations

It is up to the wellness coach to provide clear terms of reference in the contract and establish clear objectives from the beginning, so that both parties know what to expect. You need to:

- discuss with the client the parameters of the wellness coaching relationship

- reach agreement about what is appropriate in the relationship and what is not, what is and is not being offered, and about the client's and wellness coach's responsibilities

- determine whether there is an effective match between your coaching methods and the needs of the prospective client

- ensure the client has signed the Wellness Coaching Agreement.

Inside tip

Some clients might not know what wellness coaching is, so you will need to explain. I would suggest you work out a short blurb which you can adapt to suit. Here are couple of examples to kick-start you:

1. Wellness coaching is about encouraging you to change aspects of your life that are unhealthy; for example, changing dietary habits, getting more exercise or smoking cessation. Even more important, I work with you to understand how your present lifestyle contributes to those behaviours, and what can be done to change your behaviour so you achieve better health.

2. As your wellness coach, I work with you to help you improve all areas of wellness including fitness, nutrition, weight, stress, health and management of the life issues that impact wellness.

Step 2: Move onto co-creating the Personal Wellness Plan (PWP)

The PWP is based on the Wellness Coaching Intro-Pack and is a co-creation activity (see example at Form 4.3). Keep asking the client questions and let her lead the process. You are asking her to identify goals and the reasons for the goals. Clarify what the different interventions are and share your rationale of why you are suggesting certain strategies. It is the client's responsibility to accept, decline or adapt any suggestions you make. Work this intervention checklist against each goal the client wants to engage with:

- meditation and mindfulness
- bodywork interventions, e.g. massage, reflexology
- whole medical interventions, e.g. Ayurveda, chiropractic, homeopathy, naturapathic medicine, osteopathy and traditional Chinese medicine
- mindbody interventions, e.g. aromatherapy, art therapy, autosuggestion, flower remedies, Feldenkrais method, yoga, hypnotherapy, metamorphic technique, journalling, meditation, music therapy, Reiki, self-hypnosis, trager approach, visualization
- biologically based therapy, e.g. herbal therapy, diet/food, dietary supplements, exercise, naturopathy
- manipulative and body-based methods, e.g. active isolate stretching, acupressure, Alexander technique, bodywork, chiropractic, cranio sacral therapy, Feldenkrais method, manual lymphatic drainage, martial arts, massage therapy, medical acupuncture, metamorphic technique, myofascial release, osteopathy, polarity therapy, reflex point therapy, rolfing, shiatsu, trager approach
- energy therapy, e.g. medical qigong, Reiki, shiatsu, therapeutic touch
- spiritual coaching
- talking therapies, e.g. counselling, psychotherapy, hypnotherapy
- relaxation coaching, e.g. progressive muscular relaxation, autogenic coaching, breathing techniques
- cognitive behavioural coaching
- interpersonal coaching, e.g. communication skills, anger management, assertiveness coaching
- self-management coaching, e.g. anxiety management, motivation management, increasing self-esteem, managing change
- lifestyle interventions, e.g. smoking cessation, time management, work/life balance, exercise and activity, nutrition, environmental stress, ergonomics.

A PWP not only provides clients with a clear idea of what they are going to do and how they are going to do it, but gives the sessions a focus. If appropriate, clients can have a copy of the PWP at the beginning of the coaching relationship. The PWP can be used to set a framework and record progress. Wellness coaching is an organic process. Where a client wants to be at the start of the process will often change as the process unfolds, giving rise to new goals. There may be occasions when the PWP needs to be renegotiated during the coaching period. This is perfectly acceptable and can often be a useful way of refocusing on objectives. This step may take up the body of one session. If it doesn't, you can begin to work on an issue from the PWP.

Inside tip

You may already be working with your client in a therapeutic capacity, in which case the opening session has already occurred and you have a working relationship with your client. However, if you want to integrate wellness coaching into the sessions, you will need to introduce the concept; as such, this becomes the initial wellness coaching session.

Step 3: Agree frequency and number of sessions

Suggest the sessions are at least fortnightly in order to be effective and keep the momentum going. However, especially at the beginning of the process, once a week may be more desirable until the objectives are clearly sorted out. The frequency of the sessions can be decreased as the client begins to require less intensive coaching.

There is no ideal number of meetings, as each individual's needs are different. Some clients like to agree a set amount of sessions.

If you are providing face-to-face sessions, you might want to allow one-hour for the wellness coaching, or you might want to blend your time with a therapy, for example reflexology, therefore making the session longer.

Step 4: Negotiate goals and tasks

Based on Step 2, summarize the content of the session and negotiate tasks for the client to work on between sessions using the Client Action Plan Sheet (see example at Form 4.4).

Ensure that the client's goals are SMART (specific, measurable, achievable, realistic and time-bound). Leave time to ask if the client envisages any problem with the goals. It is important that problems are identified and possible solutions discussed. Be mindful of long-term goals which need dolly-step tasks to move them forward between sessions.

You may want to give your clients a copy of the Session Preparation Sheet (Form 4.5). They can complete this prior to the start of every session and either email it to you or bring it with them. This sheet details what they have achieved since the last session and gives both of you some idea of the focus for the forthcoming session.

Always sum up progress or areas covered at the end of the session using positive, upbeat language.

Step 5: Set the next appointment (and obtain your fee if your client hasn't paid up front!)

Form 4.3
Personal Wellness Plan

Wellness coaching solution checklist

Goals I would like to work on	Suggested intervention
1.	
2.	
3.	
4.	
5.	
6.	

Form 4.4
Client Action Plan Sheet

Goal	Steps needed	Resources needed	Date completed

Form 4.5
Session Preparation Sheet

Date:

To get the most from our next wellness coaching session, it is best to spend several minutes preparing for it. Please email or post me a copy of this sheet before our session.

What I have accomplished since our last session:

The goal I would like to work towards in my next wellness coaching session:

Challenges I am facing right now:

How I want to use my wellness coach today and what I want to get out of this call/session:

How to facilitate ongoing wellness sessions

Your first wellness coaching session is under your belt. Broadly speaking, each ongoing session should have a check-in, main body and conclusion. Again, I don't want to be prescriptive in how you deliver ongoing sessions, but these steps may give you focus.

Step 1: Check in

Use this time to check in: How has the client done with the agreed tasks? If you're delivering a one-hour wellness coaching session, allow around ten minutes for this.

Step 2: Main body of session

Based on the PWP or any relevant wellness issue your clients have brought to the session, use this time to coach your clients. Within ten minutes, ask clients what they would like to be the outcome from this session. Keep clients moving towards self-awareness and possible solutions related to the desired outcome, as you work towards the last 15 minutes of the session. Facilitate your clients. Let them come up with possible solutions. Be as non-directive as possible and don't spoon feed them. If there are genuine gaps in the solution process, you might want to drip-feed them ideas. Coach them in any relevant skills.

INTEGRATING LIMITING CLIENT MINDSETS

Refer to back to Module 2 and how you might work with clients' limiting mindsets. You can tell if clients hve a mindset that is less then helpful. For example, they might not elucidate or expand on your questioning, or they might find problems with each possible solution that presents itself. If clients become uncomfortable, they can put up barriers by deflecting your questions and responding through verbal diarrhoea or jabbering about unrelated subjects.

If a difficult area of discussion presents itself, be guided by the client. If she want to dive in and get to grips with it – follow her. A useful tactic is to visit the subject alongside the client, then move away to another area of (related) discussion before coming back again to the difficult issue for another visit.

UNCLEAR MOTIVATION

The client may appear stuck, not because of a limiting mindset but because her motivation is unclear. Refer back to Module 3 for further guidance.

BALANCING BETWEEN COACHING AND COUNSELLING

It can be all too easy for wellness coaching to slip into a potential counselling session. If you are a counsellor, decide how the boundaries work for you. If you are not a counsellor, recognize when the boundaries have been crossed and what you are going to do about it; for example, refer the client on or focus the client on the coaching objectives only.

DEALING WITH EMOTIONS

Coaching students often ask me how much they should let their clients explore their emotions. The clients' emotions are as important as any other part of their lives and are part of psychological wellness. However, if you get a sense that the client is having substantial difficulties in self-managing his emotions, you may need to recommend counselling. If the client needs to explore emotional content and is obviously self-managing reasonably well – and you feel comfortable in supporting him, go for it. It is about degree. If sessions are often dominated by distress that does not give way to clearer thought, improved sense of well-being and commitment to new actions, this may be an indication of deeper therapeutic issues or that the individual is stuck and requires a different kind of help. Don't stay there for the duration, but allow some time and space for the client to unload and make cognitive connections. Then when the time seems right, move the client gently and firmly forward.

Inside tip

Knowing when a client should be referred for therapy is a difficult issue because the client may not welcome this suggestion, nor take it up. This is one of the reasons why coaches need to be in supervision: to discuss their concerns as well as getting reassurance and guidance. These times may not often arise, but the wellness coach does need to recognize that there may be occasions when referral is the wisest thing to do.

CLIENT NOT ENGAGING WITH TASKS

It may be that the client isn't engaging fully in the tasks, either in the body of the session or as part of agreed homework. This needs to be addressed during the session. Use immediacy, for example 'You don't seem to be too keen on this task. Why do you think this might be?' or 'You have agreed to completing a mood journal for the past couple of sessions, but you say there hasn't been the time to complete it. How would it be if we had a chat about this?'

CLIENT REVEALING UNLAWFUL BEHAVIOUR

Another popular question from students is supposing a coaching client reveals a humdinger about something she's done. What should the coach do? Several times, I've been in the situation where a therapy or coaching client has revealed something unlawful. First, endeavour not to react. Inside you might be all of a dither, but maintain positive body language and ensure your language is non-judgemental. You can choose to limit the client's comments by not asking questions. Or you may need to know more. Be mindful about *why* you want to know more. Is it for your benefit or the client's? Will knowing more be helpful to the client? If you decide to know more, be mindful of not falling into the client's distress or moving into a place of judgement. I would strongly suggest you take the issue to supervision and discuss it with your supervisor before taking substantial action.

DEALING WITH A LACK OF CONFIDENCE OR LOW SELF-ESTEEM

Sometimes a client is full of vim and vigour and genuinely wants to change and move on. However, you get the impression of an underlying issue with low self-esteem. Until this issue is dealt with and the positives strengthened, it might be difficult for some clients to truly move on. Deal with one layer at a time in an organic fashion. Don't be too keen to get to the desired outcome. In order to for the desired outcome to be truly workable, you may need to strengthen the steps in getting there.

USING SELF-DISCLOSURE

When training students in coaching skills, I often see the student confused about when to use self-disclosure to the client. This technique can be incredibly useful, or it can bring a session to a skidding halt. Self-disclosure needs to be relevant to the client – not you. If you self-disclose because it makes you feel or look good, that is the wrong reason. Self-disclosure needs to happen because it is likely to move the client on. Sometimes the self-disclosure from the coach can reassure the client that the coach truly understands. It can build rapport. The comments need to be brief and pertinent to the client's situation. Following disclosure, immediately link back to the client's journey.

WORKING WITH CULTURAL DIFFERENCES

Cultural differences arise from different origins: birthplace, nationality, ethnicity, family status, gender, age, language, education, profession or place of work, physical condition, sexual orientation or religion. These differences can result in higher or lower levels of perceived performance. When coaching someone from a different culture, be open with yourself and your client about the implications of the cultural differences, and commit to building shared values and expectations in relation to wellness coaching.

REFRAMING USING METAPHORS

Reframing is where clients say something which you present in another way to help them understand from another perspective what they are uncertain about.

It can be useful to use metaphor and analogy to help to illustrate a point or paint a verbal picture:

Client: I would like more time at the weekend. More space for myself.

Coach: How might that be achieved?

Client: I could maybe do domestic tasks on a Saturday and leave Sunday free.

Coach: So having your Sunday free would be like creating an open space for yourself?

Client: Yes.

Coach: How might you like to use this open space?

The wellness coach needs to facilitate the metaphor process (which is similar to using guided imagery) and to offer insight that help the client gain awareness, make changes and achieve results.

Step 3: Conclusion

Approximately 15 minutes from the session's end, give a time warning and summarize the main body of the session. Use the rest of the time to facilitate the client completing the Client Action Plan based on the solutions which have arisen during the main body of the session. Set the date for next session.

How to coach a skill

Everybody has heard the old saying that a picture paints a thousand words. Coaching a new skill is a very important component of wellness coaching, and you need to be aware of some important guidelines when coaching others.

Your demonstration

Sometimes you might need to demonstrate a skill, such as breathing techniques, to your client. Use these tips to ensure the client understands what you expect of them.

PREPARATION

- Highlight the relevance to the client of the skill and talk through the main points. Keep your explanations simple and brief. Don't give your client more than two or three main points at a time. Avoid pointing out things *not* to do, as this will only overload the client.

DEMONSTRATION

- It might be appropriate to break the skill in to separate components for the purpose of the demonstration – but in any case, demonstrate the complete skill at normal speed before and at the end.

- Explain things fully. Don't just coach the technique – explain why you are doing something and how it will be used.

Client practice

After your demonstration, clients need time to practise the skill. Be positive and supportive when you notice errors. Use the 'sandwich technique' when giving feedback; for example, 'That was good, John. However, you would get even better results if you made the out-breath longer. Let's try again and see how it might help you.'

How to end the wellness coaching relationship

Because the wellness coaching process can be intense, endings can make some clients uncomfortable. Too abrupt an ending can lead to clients feeling abandoned. Too much dependency doesn't encourage empowerment, which is what wellness coaching is about.

Prepare the ground for ending on the penultimate session. Remind the client that the process is coming to an end. It is a good time for you both to reflect on the process and achievements. Issues, which might be worth looking at, include:

- List the original reasons for coming into wellness coaching.

- How were these reasons met by the end of the coaching relationship?

- What did the client gain from the sessions?

- What new needs have been identified?

- What might be the client's next step following the end of the coaching relationship?

- What can the client do longer term to maintain his wellness?

Ensure the last session is upbeat. Summarize successes. Let the client know how you have experienced the sessions (in a positive way). Co-create future wellness opportunities with the client. You may agree to speak on the telephone on occasion following the end of the process, or you might want to arrange a follow-up session, perhaps in three months' time. It might be a good idea to have a client evaluation sheet which not only provides valuable insight into how you can improve your service but will also provide testimonials!

CPD task sheet

This is your Continuing Professional Development (CPD) task sheet which summarizes key module points and offers you the opportunity to engage with tasks to deepen your learning.

Module summary

- An introduction pack allows the client time to reflect on what they want from wellness coaching, saves time in the first session and allows you to prepare in advance.

- Working with body language, effective questioning and active listening are pivotal to the wellness coaching process.

- Building rapport is the underpinning requirement to building an effective wellness coaching relationship.

- Providing constructive feedback and accepting client feedback helps to build rapport.

- The structure of sessions is important to client security and your presentation of professionalism.

Your tasks

1. How can you build on your existing health questionnaire to add to the Wellness Coaching Intro-Pack?

2. What are your body language, questioning and listening techniques like? How can you improve them?

3. How do you build client rapport?

4. Reflect on how you provide and receive feedback?

5. How might you improve the structure of your sessions?

Cognitive Behavioural Coaching

By the end of the module, you will have explored:

- Defining cognitive behavioural coaching
- The eight-step process to using CBC in wellness coaching
- Step 1: Setting the scene for CBC
- Step 2: Problem identification
- Step 3: Choices and consequences
- Step 4: Goal selection
- Step 5: Exploring and challenging faulty thinking
- Step 6: Decision-making and action planning
- Step 7: Implementation
- Step 8: Evaluation

Caution!

Cognitive behavioural coaching in the context of wellness coaching skills is *not* a substitute for treatment by a qualified cognitive behavioural therapist who has undergone four years of training.

The techniques presented in this module are designed to be used with caution. If you think your client has mental health problems, is emotionally distressed or cognitively impaired, you need to refer that person to a GP or to the British Association for Behavioural and Cognitive Psychotherapies (a list can be found at babcp.com).

If you intend to use cognitive behavioural coaching to any great depth within your wellness coaching practice, it is advised you take further training.

Defining cognitive behavioural coaching

A key skill within wellness coaching is cognitive behavioural coaching (CBC). CBC is derived from the principles and practice of cognitive behaviour therapy (CBT). CBT evolved out of Joseph Wolpe's behaviour therapy in the 1950s (Wolpe 1969), which gradually combined with elements of Aaron Beck's Cognitive Therapy (CT) (Beck 1975), Albert Ellis' Rational-Emotive Behaviour Therapy (REBT) (Ellis 1957) and a number of other influences from the cognitive approaches to psychotherapy which appeared in the 1950s and 1960s.

Cognitive behavioural approaches emphasize that how we react to events is largely determined by our views of them, not by the events themselves. Through re-evaluating unhelpful mindsets, we can implement alternative viewpoints that may be more effective in aiding problem-solving and changing behaviour.

CBC is used with non-clinical groups and can be utilized within wellness coaching most effectively. CBC does not seek to give clients the answers, but through a collaborative process helps them reach their own solutions. Drawing on and adding to clients' existing skills, CBC helps clients to build self-reliance and confidence in managing change in their lives.

CBC is time-limited, goal-directed and focused on the here and now, similar to wellness coaching. The past may be referred to in order to facilitate understanding. The main objective of wellness coaching is to help clients develop action plans for change and increase self-awareness so that they can become their own wellness coach (with occasional boosters from you).

CBC is founded on the understanding that feelings and behaviours are directly affected by the way people think. These faulty patterns of thinking give rise to emotional distress; by altering these unrealistic thought patterns, clients can reduce emotional distress.

CBC can help clients change how they think (cognitive) and what they do (behaviour). The process can help clients make sense of overwhelming problems by breaking them down into smaller parts. As shown in Figure 5.1, these parts are:

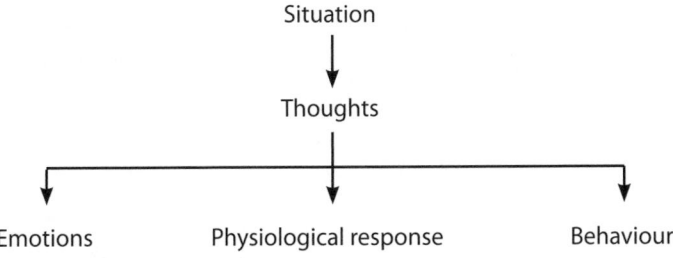

Figure 5.1 The cognitive behavioural flow chart

Each of these areas can affect the others. How you think about a problem can affect how you feel physically and emotionally. Your interpretation can also alter your behavioural response.

An example

There are helpful and unhelpful ways of reacting to most situations, depending on how you think about them.

Situation: You've had a slight falling out with a friend and who had made arrangements to call you today, and as yet, she hasn't called.

Table 5.1 Unhelpful and helpful responses to a situation		
	Unhelpful	**Helpful**
Thoughts	Mary is ignoring me. She doesn't like me any more.	I know Mary was meeting her parents from the airport today. I wonder if there has been a delay in the flight.
Feelings	Rejected, unhappy.	Concern for Mary and her parents.
Physical	Low energy.	None. Feeling comfortable.
Behaviour	Sulking.	Phone up to ensure all is well.

Table 5.1 shows that the same situation has led to two different results. How you think has affected how you felt and what you did. The unhelpful route led to negativity. The helpful route was more comfortable.

CBC can help clients to break unhelpful circles of thinking, feelings and behaviour. When they see the separate parts of the sequence, they can change them and change the way they feel and behave. CBC aims to get clients to a point where they can do it themselves and work out their own ways of tackling issues.

Using the ABC model

Albert Ellis (1962) developed what he called the 'ABC model' which describes the sequence of events that ultimately lead to our experienced feelings. He recommends that people break down their experience into these three areas in order to discover if distortions or 'irrational beliefs' are present.

'A' IS THE ACTIVATING EVENT

Activating events are the experiences we encounter. These events are described in factual, objective terms; for example, 'I stay late at work until 7:00 PM on most weekdays.'

'B' IS THE BELIEF

This is where you access faulty thinking, images and beliefs.

'C' IS THE CONSEQUENT EMOTIONS

The resulting feelings experienced as a result of our interpretation of the event. Albert Ellis suggests that people differ with regard to their feelings associated with events, solely due to the fact that they have different interpretations (1962). Consequences might include:

- First the distressing emotions, e.g. anger, anxiety, depression.
- Then the physiological symptoms, e.g. sweating, palpitations.
- Finally the behaviour. Usually linked to emotion:
  - Anxiety emotions tend to be accompanied by avoidance or defensive behaviour.
  - Depression tends to be accompanied by inactivity and withdrawal.
  - Anger tends to be accompanied by overt or muted aggressive behaviour.

For example, imagine two people are made redundant; one sinks into depression and apathy while the other finds another job within a month. If emotions are a product of experience only, why did only one become depressed and remain inactive? If emotions were caused solely by events, both people in the example would have resorted to depression. Albert Ellis would argue that the two people appraised the provocation in different ways. Consider four possible emotional outcomes of the same event in Table 5.2.

Table 5.2 Four ways to appraise the same event		
Activating event	**Belief**	**Consequent emotions**
I am made redundant.	I'm a loser.	Depression
I am made redundant.	They're picking on me.	Hostility, anger
I am made redundant.	I'll never get another job.	Anxiety, panic
I am made redundant.	I'll get a better job that is more satisfying.	Excited

This illustration suggests that our emotions are largely dependent on how we evaluate ourselves as demonstrated by our behavioural response to events that happen to us, the actions of others and our underlying beliefs. We create a basic understanding of ourselves and the world around us based on our experience and learned responses. Therefore, we differ with regard to our styles of thinking. Some engage with negative interpretations and react with depression. Others see provocation in everything and react angrily. Others are able to assess most situations in a balanced manner and seem more satisfied with life.

Inside tip

When I use the ABC model, I change it around a little.

- We identify the activating event (A).
- Then I ask for the emotions (C), as these are normally quite accessible for the client. Then I ask for the physiological and the behavioural.
- I leave (B) until last. Often clients will come up with thoughts as part of (C). If they don't, I ask them to tell me more about the emotions. This always gives rise to the thoughts.

In CBC, clients need to pay attention to automatic thoughts and recognize those which are faulty. There are a number of techniques which can be easily implemented when faulty thoughts are identified, so that realistic interpretations can be discovered.

The eight-step process to using CBC in wellness coaching

Presenting clients with a problem-solving model helps work things through in a structured and systematic way. Wasik (1984) proposed a seven-step problem-solving sequence and accompanying questions that people can ask themselves at each step:

Table 5.3 Wasik's seven-step problem-solving sequence		
1	Problem identification	What is the concern?
2	Goal selection	What do I want?
3	Generation of alternatives	What can I do?
4	Consideration of consequences	What might happen?
5	Decision-making	What is my decision?
6	Implementation	Now do it!
7	Evaluation	Did it work?

I've taken this seven-step sequence of CBC and adapted it to an eight-step sequence for wellness coaching:

Table 5.4 Adapted eight-step problem-solving sequence		
1	Setting the scene for CBC	What is the CBC process? How can it help me?
2	Problem identification	What aspect of my wellness do I want to change?
3	Choices and consequences	What choices do I have? What might happen if I choose this or that?
4	Goal selection	What do I want my wellness goal to be?

Table 5.4 Adapted eight-step problem-solving sequence *cont.*		
5	Exploring and challenging faulty thinking	Identifying faulty thinking Consequences of staying with faulty thinking Self-disputing process Effective reduction of distress (or referral)
6	Decision-making and action planning	What is my decision?
7	Implementation	Now do it!
8	Evaluation	How did it work for me? What can I change?

Here's an example process if it goes well:

Table 5.5 Positive example of the eight-step problem-solving sequence		
1	Setting the scene for CBC	What is the CBC process? How can it help me?
2	Problem identification	What aspect of my wellness do I want to change? *I work full time, have a child under six, have a home to look after and would like to have more time to pamper myself.*
3	Choices and consequences	What choices do I have? What might happen if I choose this or that? *I can ask my husband to look after Joey one evening or one Saturday a month so I can go for a treatment. (He's tired after working all day. I don't think it's right to make his day longer. He needs his Saturdays.)* *I could work from home one Friday a month. Maybe I could squeeze something in then. (Supposing there was a load of work – nothing would get a look in.)*

4	Goal selection	What do I want my wellness goal to be? *I want to have time for a massage once a month.*
5	Exploring and challenging faulty thinking	Identifying faulty thinking *There is no time for a massage.* Consequences of staying with faulty thinking *Feeling resentful and stressed* Self-disputing process *There could be time, if I really thought about it. My husband is more tired in the evening, so that probably isn't a good time for him. If I went for a massage on a Saturday, he could have a lay in. I would only be away a couple of hours; he could take care of Joey then.* Effective reduction of distress (or referral) *I'm relieved to have some time to myself.*
6	Decision-making and action planning	What is my decision? *I'm going ask my husband how he feels about looking after Joey for a couple of hours on a Saturday once a month so I can have a massage.*
7	Implementation	Now do it! *My husband was fine about taking care of Joey; it gives him some quality time with him. I have found a massage therapist who works Saturdays and booked an appointment.*
8	Evaluation	How did it work for me? What can I change? *The massage was wonderful. An oasis each month and something to look forward to. Husband's over the moon at having a go at Joey's train set! I've booked for next month.*

Sometimes during the coaching process, clients may become emotionally distressed (around Step 5), thereby lessening their ability to focus on the issue. If this emotional interference occurs, the wellness coach can employ the ABCDE sequence of emotional management (Neenan and Dryden 2000):

A: Activating event. Stop working on the solution chosen at Step 5.

B: Identify distress-producing **B**eliefs, e.g. I'll never sort this out.

C: **C**onsequences: Identify distressing emotions and behaviour, e.g. anger and agitation.

D: Engage in self-**D**isputing process, e.g. 'I'll never sort this out' becomes 'Change isn't always quick and easy. If it takes a little longer, it doesn't matter.'

E: **E**ffective reduction in anger and agitation enabling the person to return to working with their proposed solution at Step 5.

It isn't helpful to follow the eight-step model when the client is emotionally upset. When clients' emotional distress has been alleviated, they can resume following the problem-solving model. If there is no alleviation in their emotional state, a referral to a clinical therapist may indicated. Here's an example process when it doesn't go well!

	Table 5.6 Challenging example of the eight-step problem-solving sequence	
1	Setting the scene for CBC	What is the CBC process? How can it help me?
2	Problem identification	What aspect of my wellness do I want to change? *I hate the fact that I'm always tired. I work full time, have a child under six, have a home to look after and never have any time for going to pamper myself. I always seem to be doing things for other people. I'm really angry about it.*
3	Choices and consequences	What choices do I have? What might happen if I choose this or that? *I can ask my husband to look after Joey in the evening, but he's never around.* *I could work from home on a Friday. But I'd only end up doing the housework!* *I could get a part-time job. But there's nothing out there. Who'd have me, anyway?*

4	Goal selection	What do I want the outcome to be? *I don't want to feel stressed. There's too much happening. I want everybody to go away.*
5	Exploring and challenging faulty thinking	Identifying faulty thinking *My husband's never around.* *There's too much housework to do.* *I've no money to pay for treats.* Consequences of staying with faulty thinking *Feeling resentful and stressed. Not bothering to change anything.* Self-disputing process *It's hopeless. Nothing ever changes. I've got to keep working this hard to keep the money coming in.* Effective reduction of distress (or referral) *Resentment and stress.*
6	Decision-making and action planning	What is my decision? *I can't change anything.*
7	Implementation	Now do it! *I can't do it. I've got no support. No one is helping me.*
8	Evaluation	How did it work for me? What can I change? *I'm stuck with it and feel awful about everything.*

CBC is particularly useful when a client has got stuck in their processes. If, for example, wellness needs have been identified but the client is resistant to moving onto setting goals, you could use CBC in exploring the whys and wherefores. Another time to use CBC is when a client has agreed to negotiated tasks but isn't engaging with them in practice. Clients will fully engage in wellness coaching when they are motivated. Sometimes the motivations are blurred and therefore prevent clients from getting the best from the coaching process. CBC can help uncover beliefs and motivations and, where appropriate, reframe them.

Step 1: Setting the scene for CBC
Introducing CBC

You can introduce CBC into a wellness coaching session formally or informally. As we go through the eight-step process, we'll accompany a fictitious client called Tom.

A formal introduction might mean a deliberate explanation, for example:

> I'd like to introduce a technique to you called cognitive behaviourial coaching or CBC for short. Let me explain how this technique could help you move past some of your blocks you're experiencing about this particular wellness issue.
>
> Think of a triangle. At the apex we have our thought processes. Our thought processes influence our emotions and our behaviours. Our thoughts can sometimes be faulty, and this can contribute to distressing emotions or inappropriate behaviour.

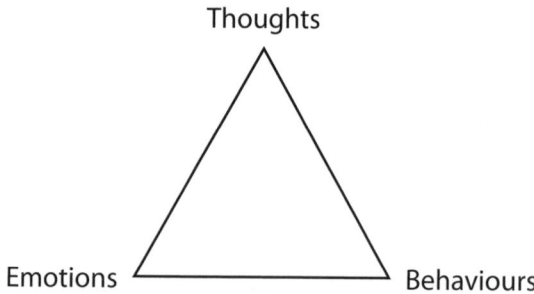

Figure 5.2 The links between thoughts, emotions and behaviours

Not every thought is faulty. We have many thoughts that are constructive and helpful. We also have thoughts, which although uncomfortable, are nevertheless true. However, there are times when we have what is called faulty thinking which holds us back from making constructive changes.

Inside tip

I tend to ask clients at this point, without being patronizing, if they understand the difference between thoughts and feelings. I ask them to give me their immediacy of both. Do a quickie: How are you feeling right now? What are you thinking right now? How are you physiologically right now?

Once I know that they know the difference (many don't), I move onto the Identifying Common Cognitive Errors sheet, Table 5.7. I ask clients to read it and to tell me what, if any, scenarios they identify with. Most people can identify several.

I then move onto a fresh sheet of paper with the headings:

EVENT   FEELING   THOUGHT   PHYSIOLOGICAL   BEHAVIOUR

I ask clients to think of an event in the past week that has caused them some distress, and I work through the form with them. Then I ask them to think of another event and they fill in another sheet themselves. This particular exercise prepares them for the ABC model.

The informal introduction to CBC is where you seamlessly start to use the techniques without any explanation.

Is your client CBC ready?

Before using this technique, ensure your client is CBC ready. Don't use CBC if your client has mental health problems, is emotionally distressed or cognitively impaired.

Inside tip

Thoughts are like quicksilver. There, then gone. We are constantly thinking, and most of the time we are unaware of the thoughts and more aware of the emotions. In order for CBC to work for your clients, they need to practise it every day. Every time faulty thinking is identified, it needs to be modified. If faulty thinking is ignored, old ways are strengthened. However, awareness and practice strengthens a new way of thinking, which then eventually becomes automatic. If your client isn't prepared to work at it, CBC isn't going to produce results.

Identifying Common Cognitive Errors

Aaron Beck (1975) identifies common errors in Table 5.7.

Table 5.7 Beck's Common Cognitive Errors	
All-or-nothing thinking	Placing experiences in one of two opposite categories
Over-generalizing	Making sweeping inference based on a single incident
Discounting the positive	Deciding that if a good thing has happened, it couldn't have been very important
Jumping to conclusions	Focusing on one aspect of a situation when judging
Mind-reading	Believing one knows what another person is thinking with little or no evidence
Fortune-telling	Believing one knows what the future holds while ignoring other possibilities
Magnifying/ minimizing	Evaluating the importance of a negative event or the lack of evidence of a positive event in a distorted manner
Emotional reasoning	Believing that something must be true because it feels true
Making 'should' statements	Telling oneself one should do (or should have done) something when it is more accurate to say that one would like to do (or wishes one had done) the preferred thing
Inappropriate blaming	Using a label, e.g. 'stupid' or 'useless driver' to describe a behaviour and then imputing all the meanings the label carries

Using effective questioning

When eliciting possible cognitive errors with a wellness coaching client, you may find these types of questions useful to ask:

- Is this thought logical?
- Where is the evidence for your belief?

- Is your belief realistic?
- Would your friends and colleagues agree with your ideas?
- Does everybody share your attitude? If not, why not?
- Are you expecting yourself or others to be perfect as opposed to fallible human beings?
- What makes the situation so terrible?
- Will it seem this bad in one, three or six months' time?
- Are you fortune-telling with little evidence that the worst case scenario will actually happen?
- If you 'can't stand it' or 'can't bear it', what will really happen?
- Are you concentrating on your own (or others') weaknesses and neglecting strengths?
- Are you agonizing about how you think things should be instead of dealing with them as they are?
- Where is this thought or attitude getting you?
- How is your belief helping you to attain your goals?
- Is your belief goal- and problem-solving focused?
- If a friend made a similar mistake, what might you say to them?
- Are you thinking in all-or-nothing terms? Is there any middle ground?
- Are you labelling yourself, somebody or something else? Is this logical and a fair thing to do?
- Just because a problem has occurred does it mean that you/they/it are 'stupid', a 'failure', 'useless' or 'hopeless'?
- Are you placing rules on yourself or others, e.g. 'should' or 'must'? If so, are they proving helpful and constructive?
- Are you taking things too personally?
- Are you blaming others unfairly just to make yourself (temporarily) feel better?

Explaining the importance of negotiated tasks

You will need to explain the importance of wellness tasks which are negotiated during the session and completed by the client between sessions. Wellness coaching is a lifestyle change opportunity; therefore, the learning moves outside of the comfort zone of the session and into real life.

Step 2: Problem identification

You've set the scene for CBC. The client should understand the process now.

The next step is to ask the client for problem identification: What aspect of their wellness do they want to change? This has been partially identified at the Wellness Coaching Intro-Pack stage. From this, you would have co-created a PWP with the client. Although the PWP is the basis of the wellness coaching process, it is likely to organically change.

Let's get back to Tom who initially might have identified the following issues to work on:

1. not bringing work home, therefore having more quality time with family

2. not drinking so much alcohol

3. increasing activity levels.

Each issue needs to be explored as to the problems they cause and why the client wants to change. For the sake of this exercise, we'll focus on the first issue: his not wanting to bring work home in order to have family time. We might want to ask him why he feels the need to bring work home, what kind of pressure he is under in relation to work, what expectations does the client have of himself in relation to work, how the workload affects other areas of his life, etc. Move the client from a general problem to specifics; in our example, this might be:

- I need to bring the work home because I keep getting interrupted at work. If I don't get it all done, they will think I can't do my job.
  There is an underlying problem of constant interruptions at work. Tom believes that his bosses will think he can't do his job.

- Two members of our department have been made redundant already, and if I can't keep up, I might be next.
  Tom believes he can't keep up and that he might be made redundant because others will see this too.

- I don't have a lunch-break anymore, sometimes I stay late and often I bring work home.
  There is the behaviour of not having a lunch-break, of staying late and of taking work home.

Tom has identified that he doesn't want to bring work home, the pay-off (or motivation) being more quality time with his family. Specifically, we can see that Tom has behaviours of not taking a lunch-break, of staying late and of taking work home. His beliefs include: the bosses will think he can't do his job, he can't keep up, he might be made redundant. There is an external problem of work interruptions.

Step 3: Choices and consequences

Tom has identified his problem. We now look at generating solutions to the identified problem of not taking a lunch-break, staying late and taking work home, and to explore the possible consequences of these solutions.

Left- and right-brain creativity

If you can coach your clients to use their creative abilities in balance with logical planning and evaluation, they will be better placed to find solutions to problems. There are a number of processes to go through to channel creativity into productivity, as seen at Figure 5.3.

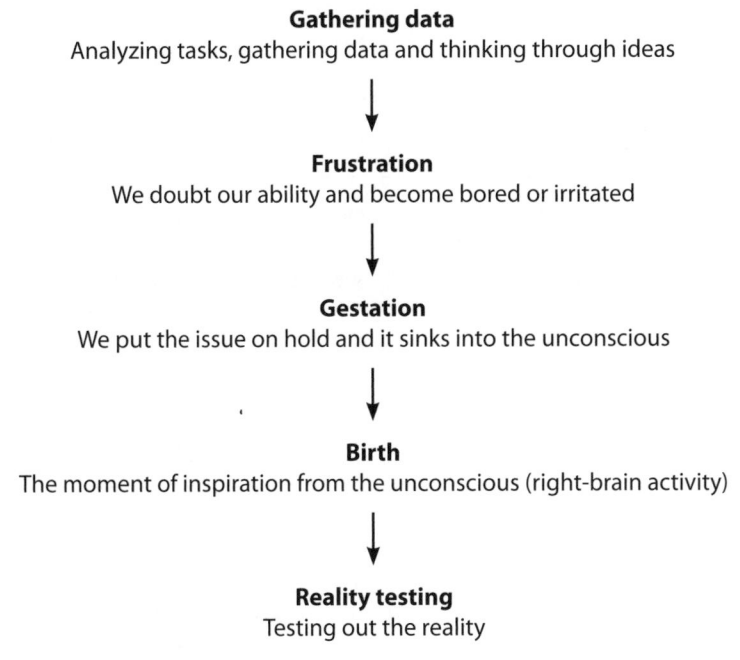

Gathering data
Analyzing tasks, gathering data and thinking through ideas

Frustration
We doubt our ability and become bored or irritated

Gestation
We put the issue on hold and it sinks into the unconscious

Birth
The moment of inspiration from the unconscious (right-brain activity)

Reality testing
Testing out the reality

Figure 5.3 The creative flow chart

The left hemisphere of the brain is almost always larger than the right hemisphere, and each hemisphere performs a different function. One of the most important advances in the study of the brain occurred in the 1960s and 1970s when Roger Sperry of the California Institute of Technology and his team of researchers developed the understanding that the human brain consists of two hemispheres (see Table 5.8), each of which controls different processes (Sperry, Hubel and Wiesel 1981).

Balanced creativity is utilizing the right side of the brain in the 'birthing' process, and making those ideas a reality through left-brain activities. Coaching skills for left- and right-brain balance is helpful to your client's wellness development.

Table 5.8 Two hemisphere process	
Left brain	**Right brain**
linear thought	the ability to see patterns linking ideas
verbalizes to describe	uses gestures or pictures to describe
logical	constructs geometric and perspective images
breaks down the whole into parts	puts parts together to form a whole
limited spatial sense	good spatial and pattern sense
uses symbols in representation	sees things as they are
good numerical sense	limited numerical sense
good time sense	limited time sense
relies on fact	relies on instinct and intuition
speech-orientated	comprehends simple language
language-orientated	creative and imaginative

The creative psyche

To understand and develop inner creativity, we need to understand the psyche. Beneath the ego (perceptions of who we think we are or would like to be) is the essential Self (the unconscious) that guides and directs the body through the subconscious mind. We know that something keeps our heart pumping and lungs breathing without conscious intent. This has been called the 'subconscious'. The subconscious also houses the full potential of the psyche. When we tap this inner realm and raise the subconscious intent to conscious awareness, we get in touch with and utilize our inner creativity.

There are many ways to reach this inner creative potential. First we need to put the ego to rest temporarily. The chattering personality (or 'monkey mind') needs to be set aside for a time so that the psyche can see the light of mind. Some good methods of quieting our thoughts are:

- Meditation, which puts our brain into an alpha state, or, as we become proficient, a wakeful theta state. In this altered state, the gap will open and creative mind emerges.

- Soft focus, which is an excellent way to stop the thinking process. Soft focus your eyes through a gentle gaze on a neutral surface, e.g. a wall or ceiling. Be aware of everything around you without focusing on anything. Your peripheral vision will increase and the subconscious mind of creativity will come to the surface.

- Mindfulness is a meditative state of enhanced awareness, focused on the now. When we are mindful, our mind is less distracted and we can access and draw out our creative process.

- Controling the breath greatly aids clarity of mind. Levels of oxygen in the brain are linked to levels of serotonin, the neurotransmitter hormone that makes us awake and alert. Too much serotonin in the brain causes stress. Reduced serotonin results in relaxation and allows the brain's intuitive activities to flow smoothly. When you need to produce a more heightened state of awareness for immediate problem-solving, you can control your breathing and drop the levels of serotonin. Here are two methods for increasing brain hormonal and hemispherical balance:

  ○ One method is holding the breath momentarily between breaths. This oxygenates the brain and facilitates clarity. Deep breathing promotes alpha brain waves and relaxes the body and mind. Inhale through the nose for a count of five, hold for a beat, and then exhale through the mouth for a count of seven. Hold for a beat before inhaling once more. Continue for several cycles.

  ○ Another method is to breathe through alternating nostrils. The Chinese believe that the nostrils are an indication of hemispherical dominance. Whichever nostril you habitually breathe through can tell you which side of the brain you favour. Pinch your nostrils together across the bridge of your nose and release the right nostril. Inhale through your right nostril for a count of four. Pinch for a count of four. Release the left nostril and exhale for a count of four. Inhale through your left nostril for a count of four. Pinch for a count of four. Release the right nostril and exhale for a count of four. Repeat the cycle four times. If you practise this for about ten minutes, you will improve your mental clarity. You will also slow down your brain waves, from beta to alpha, facilitating intuitive thought.

In the case of Tom, possible solutions might include finding ways to lessen work interruptions, delegating tasks, time management and talking to his boss.

Consequences of solutions

Now Tom needs to work through the possible consequences of the solutions. Ideally the consequences are that his workload would be dealt with more efficiently, resulting in a regular lunch-break, not working late every night or not working quite so late and not taking work home. He would then have more time with his family.

When working through consequences, be realistic and identify possible problem areas and solutions. For example, in Tom's scenario, there may not be the appropriate people to delegate to or his boss might not be helpful.

Step 4: Goal selection

The problem has been identified and choices and consequences explored. Now is the time to set realistic and achievable goals based on the choices.

Effective goal-setting is a powerful technique that can yield strong returns in wellness. Your client, under your facilitation, identifies areas for change which are formulated as wellness goals. From this, you create an Action Plan from each session, with results that are SMART:

- **S**pecific
- **M**easurable
- **A**ttainable
- **R**ealistic
- **T**imebound

Planning skills

Planning is the start of the process by which you can help your client turn goals into achievements. The process helps clients to:

- take stock of their current position and identify precisely what is to be achieved
- work out the process of getting there in the most effective, efficient way

- detail precisely the who, what, when, where, why and how of achieving the goal
- consider the control mechanisms that are needed to achieve the plan and keep it on course
- evaluate whether the effort, costs and implications of achieving the plan is worth the effort
- focus on the critical factors to ensure preparation for all reasonable eventualities
- gather the resources needed
- assess the impact of the plan.

There are a number of reasons why planning doesn't happen, as shown in Table 5.9.

Table 5.9 Reasons for not planning	
Crisis management	Clients may be so embroiled in crisis management that they don't have the time to plan.
Apathy	Clients may not bother to put in the time necessary to think a plan through.
Lack of commitment/ resistance to change	Clients may not see the benefits of the planning process. They may believe that there is no need to plan, or may decide that things are OK as they are.
Bad planning experience	Clients may have had a previous bad experience with planning, where plans have been inflexible, cumbersome, or impractical.
Fear of failure	By not taking action there is little risk of failure unless a problem is urgent and pressing.

Planning is best thought of as a cycle. Once a plan has been devised, it should be evaluated for likelihood of success and unwanted consequences. If the plan produced unwanted consequences, the planning process will have to cycle back to an earlier stage or be abandoned altogether. A possible outcome of planning is that it might be best to do nothing! The stages of the planning cycle are shown in Figure 5.4.

Setting performance goals

You should take care to ensure clients set wellness goals over which they have as much control as possible. Goals based on outcomes are vulnerable to failure because of things beyond our control. If clients base their goals on personal performance or skills or knowledge to be acquired, then they can keep control over the achievement of goals.

SETTING SPECIFIC AND MEASURABLE GOALS

If clients achieve most or all conditions of a measurable goal, they can be confident and comfortable in its achievement. If they consistently fail to meet a measurable goal, then together you can adjust it or analyze the reason for failure and take appropriate action. Goals may be set unrealistically high for the following reasons:

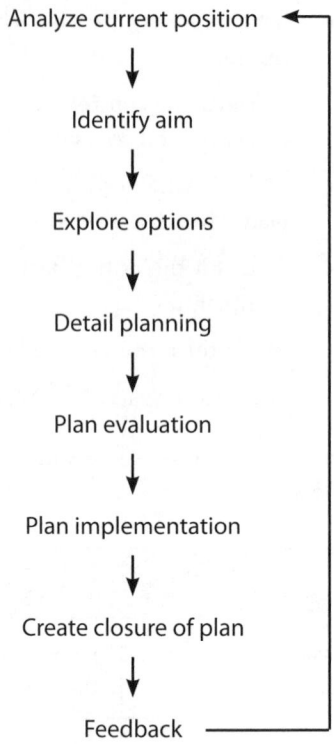

Figure 5.4 Stages of the planning cycle

- Other people such as partners, parents or media can set unrealistic goals for your client, based on what they want.

- If clients do not have a clear, realistic understanding of what they want to achieve and of the skills and knowledge necessary to get there, it is difficult to set effective and realistic goals.

- Many people base their goals on their best performance, however long ago that was. This ignores the inevitable backsliding that can occur for the best of reasons and ignores the factors that led to that best performance. It is better to set goals that raise the average performance and make it more consistent.

Alternatively goals can be set too low because of:

- Fear of failure. If clients are frightened of failure, they will not take the risks needed for optimum performance. As they apply goal-setting and see the achievement of goals, their self-confidence should increase, helping them to take bigger risks. Help clients understand that failure is a positive thing, as it shows them areas where they can improve their skills and performance.

- Taking it too easy. It is easy to take the reasons for not setting goals unrealistically high as an excuse to set them too low. If clients are not prepared to stretch themselves and work hard, they are unlikely to achieve anything of any true worth.

Setting goals at the correct level is a skill that is acquired by practice. Clients should set wellness goals that are slightly out of their immediate grasp but not so far that there is no hope of achieving them.

When you are helping clients to achieve goals, asking the following questions to help you both focus on the sub-goals that lead to their achievement:

- Is it measurable and verifiable?
- Do you understand the goal?
- Is the goal a realistic and attainable one that still represents a challenge?
- Will the result, when achieved, justify the time and resources required to achieve it?
- Is it consistent with your values and beliefs?
- What skills do you need to achieve this?
- What information and knowledge do you need?
- What help, assistance or collaboration do you need?
- What resources do you need?
- What can block your progress?

Goal-setting can go wrong for a number of reasons:

- Goals can be so vague that they are useless. If achievement cannot be measured, the clients' self-confidence will not benefit from goal-setting, nor can they observe progress towards a greater goal. Set precise, quantitative wellness-related goals.
- Goal-setting can be unsystematic, sporadic and disorganized. Goals will be forgotten, achievement of goals not be measured and feedback will not develop into new goals. Be organized and regular in the way you use goal-setting.
- Too many un-prioritized goals may be set, leading to a feeling of overload.
- The client didn't try hard enough.

- The client's technique, skills or knowledge were faulty and need to be enhanced.
- The goal set was unrealistic.

When a client has achieved a wellness goal, encourage her to take the time to enjoy the satisfaction of having achieved the goal. Help her absorb the implications of the goal achievement, and observe the progress she makes towards other goals.

Remember that wellness goals change as the client evolves. Adjust them regularly to reflect this growth. If goals stop holding any attraction, let them go. Goal-setting is a servant, not a master, and should bring your clients satisfaction and a sense of achievement.

Inside tip

The way in which you help clients set goals strongly affects their effectiveness. The following broad guidelines apply to setting effective goals:

- At the end of each session, ask clients to write down the goals on their Action Plan.
- Set a precise goal, putting in as much detail as possible.
- Where clients have several goals, give each a priority. This helps clients avoid feeling overwhelmed by too many goals, and directs their attention to the most important ones.
- Keep the goals clients want to work towards immediately small and achievable. If a goal is too large, they may feel that they are not making progress towards it.

Now your clients can create an Action Plan, as in Table 5.10. Don't assume your clients know how to complete this. Equally don't patronize them. Keep an eye on them as they go through the process for any areas of difficulty.

Let's look at Tom's Action Plan, based on his possible solutions.

Table 5.10 Tom's Action Plan			
Action	**Steps needed**	**Resources required**	**Date**
Finding ways to lessen work interruptions	Have phone calls diverted to Anna	Arrange with Anna	3 Sept.
	Work two days a week from home	Talk to boss	TBA
	Organize work space at home	Time	16 Sept.
Delegating tasks	Bert to do the monthly spreadsheets	Talk with Bert	6 Sept.
	Retail emails could have a separate email address and Anna could check them to filter out important ones	Set up with IT dept.	3 Sept.
		Talk with Anna	3 Sept.
Time management	Filter non-important meetings, find alternative ways of attending others, e.g. tele-conferencing	Talk with Geoff	4 Sept.
		Talk with Anna	3 Sept.
Talking to boss	Arrange with Mary's PA	Talk with PA	TBA

Step 5: Exploring and challenging faulty thinking

As the client goes through the process of choosing ways to implement wellness goals, it is possible that resistance to change will be met. This is when we need to explore automatic thoughts and irrational beliefs with the client, using the core coaching techniques described earlier in the book, plus a few new ones from this module.

We think or say a positive or negative automatic thought in certain situations, for example when winter time comes around and we assume we will get flu. When negative automatic thoughts control our emotional response we may ignore evidence that contradicts the thought and have an expectation of a negative outcome. For example, if we talk to someone who has a cold, we might believe we'll get a cold within the week. The automatic thoughts create an expectancy of something negative. Sometimes life is vague and can be interpreted in a variety of ways. If uncertainty is an issue for us, we may negatively evaluate the world so it agrees with our negative automatic thoughts.

Albert Ellis presented the idea that irrational beliefs are at the core of most psychological problems (Abrams 2011). Some examples of irrational beliefs are:

- If I eat all the right foods, I'll be healthy.
- If I do what is expected of me, my life will be wonderful.
- If I jog every day, I'll never get ill.
- It's a sign of weakness if I'm ill.
- I must always put others first.
- If I work all the hours God sends, I will be successful.

What makes these ideas irrational is the belief that they are always correct. Eating health foods will increase your wellness, but staying fit is not guaranteed. There are times when we do everything right, and it still doesn't hang together. This process leads some people to the conclusion that they are no good or weak, which could lead to depression or low self-esteem.

Inside tip

We have thousands of thoughts going through our mind. Not every thought is linked to a belief.

A belief is a thought we are emotionally attached to and that we make real or accept as true. We relate beliefs to practical activity. For example, you might imagine you are one of the best wellness coaches in town, but unless you believe it, you will not act as such. Beliefs conform to our faith in the possibility of the outcome.

As clients identify their automatic thoughts and irrational beliefs, we need to challenge those that seem faulty by checking their validity:

1. Question and help the client clarify their automatic thoughts. If the client finds it hard to distinguish between emotions and automatic thoughts, use the ABC framework.

2. Sift through the plethora of automatic thoughts and select the ones that are faulty. These then need to be evaluated:

   a. Focus on the faulty thought, e.g. How much do you believe this thought? How did this make you feel emotionally? How did you behave after you had this thought?

   b. Find out more about the situation associated with the faulty thought, e.g. tell me more about the situation when you spoke with, Mary, just before you had that thought.

   c. Explore how typical the faulty thought is, e.g. How often do you have this kind of thought and in what situations?

3. Identify other faulty thoughts and images in this same situation, e.g. What else goes through your mind? Any images, for example?

4. Consider solutions to the situation, e.g. What are some of the things you could do about this?

5. Explore the irrational belief that might be underlying the faulty thought, e.g. If this thought is true what would it mean to you?

When questioning faulty thoughts, Judith Beck (1995) states the following is helpful:

- What is the evidence that supports the idea and what is the evidence against the idea?

- Is there an alternative explanation?

- What is the worst that could happen and could I live through it?

- What is the effect of me believing the thought and what is the most realistic outcome?

- What should I do about it?

- What would I tell a friend if they were in the same situation?

If those thoughts or beliefs don't stand up to scrutiny, if there is little or no evidence for them, the client can choose to reframe them to more helpful ones.

Overcoming client resistance

As clients move through the wellness coaching process, their behaviour may show resistance to change. For example, they may seem closed to new experiences, respond to suggestions in a negative way and come late to or cancel appointments. They may become intensely irritated with you. They could start to feel unclear about the benefits of coaching or seem frustrated that change is not happening as fast and easily as they expected. You may find that wellness coaching clients can present a range of compensatory strategies (Beck 1995) which indicate resistance to change and represent faulty thinking, such as:

- avoiding situations that give rise to painful, negative emotions
- striving to be perfect at all times
- being overly responsible
- avoiding intimacy to protect from hurt, betrayal, rejection or abandonment
- seeking recognition
- avoiding confrontation
- being overly controlling of themselves, others and their environment
- acting in a childlike and immature manner
- desperately trying to please other people, doing and being whatever they dictate
- being highly emotional or volatile in order to attract attention
- deliberately presenting as helpless and incompetent in order to secure the help of others
- avoiding and denying all responsibility
- seeking 'love' and intimacy from any source and at any cost
- shrinking from being noticed, avoiding attention
- deliberately provoking a reaction
- abdicating control and decision-making
- being authoritarian
- pleasing only themselves, being highly independent, non-conforming and distant in relationships.

Beutler, Moleiro and Talebi (2002) identify three specific factors that contribute to levels of resistance with clients. The first relates to the subjective value placed on the area being threatened; for example, clients may resist set tasks that impinge on their perceived free time because they like to live in an unstructured way. The second relates to the proportion of freedoms being targeted; for example, clients may be willing to go to social events. However, being asked to speak to a prescribed number of people and also stay for a set period of time may, together, tip the balance and precipitate a resistant reaction.

The third factor relates to issues surrounding authority; for example, some clients may have negative associations or erroneous preconceived notions about authority figures. They may react against a wellness coach telling them what to do.

General guidelines for working with resistant clients:

- Provide client opportunities for self-directed improvement.

- Increase reliance on non-directive interventions.

- Provide suggestions and interpretations.

- De-emphasize the use of confrontational procedures.

Wellness coaching should be adapted to suit the individual by deciding on directive versus non-directive interventions.

UNCOVERING BELIEFS

To help uncover irrational beliefs, the wellness coach can use techniques, such as:

- Looking for the expression of a belief in a faulty thought, e.g. I've always had bad PMT just like my mother, and loads of my friends have it, too. All woman have PMT, I'm not alone.

- Providing the conditional clause 'If__' of an assumption and asking the client to complete it, e.g. If your cholesterol test came back high, what choices of action do you have?

- Identifying a common theme among faulty thoughts, e.g. I can't talk to strangers at a party; no one at work ever asks me for a drink after work; I clam up during family get-togethers.

- Asking the client what they think their belief is.

Sometimes the client becomes overwhelmed by his emotions and confused by a multitude of thoughts. This could be due to a core belief which takes the form of a universal rule for living, such as, I must always be completely healthy or else I am a weak person. Such a core belief generates numerous subsidiary beliefs in specific situations; for example, I have a cold, but I mustn't take time off work; or, How terrible, I have been diagnosed with varicose veins.

One way of gaining access to elusive beliefs is by vivid imagery. We might ask the client to close his eyes and imagine as vividly as possible that part of an activating event which evokes the strongest emotional reaction, such as a pre-diabetic person having a glucose test. This will stimulate the client's memory concerning his emotional reactions. While focusing on these images, the client can begin to gain access to cognitive processes below the level of awareness that cannot be easily reached through verbal dialogue. The client needs to expose himself to the event in order to access the negatively exaggerated evaluative beliefs and consequent emotional distress. The client will then be able to retrieve the elusive faulty thoughts that give rise to his distress but at the same time make use of the realistic, reframed thoughts.

Irrational beliefs tend to fall into one or other of the broad categories shown in Table 5.11.

Table 5.11 Irrational belief categories	
Helpless beliefs	**Unlovable beliefs**
I am helpless	I am worthless and valueless
I am useless	I am unlovable
I am powerless	I will be abandoned/always alone
I am vulnerable	I am bad and shameful
I am weak	I am different/defective
I am inadequate	I am not good enough (to be loved, etc.)
I am a failure	I am unacceptable
I am needy and defective	I am inferior
I am incompetent	I will (deserve to be) rejected
I am 'stuck'	I don't count

Hence a client who describes herself as ugly expects to be abandoned and/ or rejected. Or a client who believes she is basically defective (because of a disability) is likely to have an 'unlovable' belief.

In contrast, a client who works incessantly is driven by fear of failure or believes that she will under-perform or not be good enough to succeed is likely to have a 'helpless' core belief.

CHALLENGING AND REFRAMING BELIEFS

Judith Beck (1995) believes it is crucial that the client grasps the following about a core belief:

- That it is an idea and not necessarily a truth and as an idea, it can be tested.

- That the client can believe it strongly, feel it to be true and yet have it be mostly or entirely untrue.

- That it is rooted in childhood events; that it may or may not have been true at the time the client first came to believe it.

- That the client and the wellness coach working together can use a variety of strategies over time to change this idea so that the client can view himself in a more realistic way.

Once identified, we can help the client reframe the belief, as demonstrated in Table 5.12.

Table 5.12 Challenging and reframing beliefs	
I am worthless.	No one is worthless. We are all equal and have the same value. It has nothing to do with race, colour, class, background, education, career, looks, and so on.
I am inferior.	We all have strengths and weaknesses and these will differ from person to person. Thus I have strengths which others don't have and am weak in areas where others are strong.
I am helpless.	There are a lot of things I can do for myself, and there are lots of people and resources out there to help me grow and change.
I am unlovely and unlovable.	Many people like and love me. There may be some aspects of my life and I'd like to change for the better: but I also have many positive qualities and attributes.

When modifying an unhelpful belief, the wellness coach guides the client to examine the operation of the belief in specific situations, rather than dealing with the generalized belief in a global fashion. For example, 'I always get headaches' becomes 'I tend to get headaches when there is a social situation'.

Through this means, the coach can lead the client to marshal evidence which refutes the belief in specific situations.

Tools to use with the client during this stage
CHALLENGING GLOBAL THINKING

When challenging global thinking, Stephen Palmer (1997) suggests the following analogies:

- Would you throw an entire bowl of fruit away if one piece was mouldy?
- If one tissue was ripped in a box of tissues, are they all ripped?
- If one cigarette in a pack is crushed, are the rest impaired?
- Can a drop from a jug show the shape or amount within?
- Does a missing hand represent the whole body self?
- If one flower is wilted in a vase of flowers, would you discard them all?
- Does one plant name describe all the plants in your garden?
- Would you throw out all of the clothes from your wardrobe if there was one item you disliked?

THE BELIEF CONTINUUM

The use of scales for measuring the extent to which clients hold a faulty thought or irrational belief is an important technique for introducing flexibility into the thought patterns of clients, especially those who have all-or-nothing thinking. The unhelpful belief, for example 'I am a failure if I don't go to the gym five times a week', and the helpful belief, for example 'My twice weekly visits to the gym boost my energy and wellness', are first identified. The helpful belief is written at one side of a sheet of paper and a link drawn to the other side as in Figure 5.5.

My twice weekly visits to the gym boost my energy and wellness:

——————————————————————X——————————————

0 per cent   100 per cent

Figure 5.5 The belief continuum

At one end of the line is placed 0 per cent (no belief), and at the other 100 per cent (complete belief). Clients are asked to put a cross on the part of the scale they currently occupy. This will initially be towards the extreme of 0 per cent. Through a process of questioning and other techniques, it is usually possible for clients to move towards the more helpful belief.

WEIGHTING

Many people struggle with making decisions. A common task in CBC is asking clients to list and 'weigh' the advantages and disadvantages of different courses of action.

PIE CHARTS

Sometimes clients are unaware that, for example, their work and life are out of balance. A pie chart can graphically convey how clients currently use their time. They can then identify possible change that would move them towards a balanced lifestyle.

FUNCTIONAL SELF-COMPARISONS

Many clients display faulty thinking and view themselves in a negative way because of depression or low self-esteem. Such clients will tend to discount positives and will often make negative self-comparisons (either to other people or to themselves before they became ill). This technique is about challenging these comparisons.

KEEPING 'CREDIT RECORDS'

Credit records are lists of positive actions or behaviours that clients should receive credit for. Reviewing this when they feel unmotivated reminds them that they are making progress and possess many positive attributes, skills and abilities.

ROLE-PLAY

The client is helped to make a list of faulty thinking which supports the irrational belief and generates a list of reframed thoughts. The role-play begins with the client adopting the role of the unhelpful thoughts which he is currently using. The wellness coach argues against each of these in turn, using the helpful thoughts generated earlier. Once the coach has modelled the helpful role in this way, the coach and client reverse roles with the coach now becoming the devil's advocate.

GRADED TASK PERFORMANCE

Clients may confront problems that seem too big to handle. They feel overwhelmed and fear they won't cope. In order to make the task more manageable, it can be broken down into smaller, concrete chunks, which is the aim of graded task performance.

MODIFYING ACTIVATING EVENTS

A client may create a negative-activating event through poor judgement, lack of skills or blind ignorance. For example, a young lad who considers aggression basically wrong, drinks too much at parties and finds himself in aggressive brawls. If he can change the activating event by, for example, only consuming soft drinks at parties or alternate alcoholic drinks with soft drinks or water, he can then change his behaviour. If he does not allow his beliefs to change under the influence of alcohol, he can continue to behave in ways that reflect his true belief.

SOCIAL SKILLS COACHING

Sometimes a lack of knowledge hampers the client from behaving in appropriate ways; for example, a woman who was constantly criticized as a child may lack the skills and knowledge to work with criticism constructively as an adult. If such skills are taught and acquired, they can change both the client's behaviour and perception of herself.

CONTRACTING

The client makes a formal agreement with a significant other, such as a family member or work colleague, to make specific positive behavioural changes to which they both aspire, such as smoking cessation or maintaining a diet. The wellness coach emphasizes that both parties should work together as a team and remind each other of the benefits of change.

COST-BENEFIT ANALYSIS OF BEHAVIOURS/HABITS/BELIEFS

With this method the wellness coach helps clients assess the pros and cons of maintaining particular behaviours or beliefs that they wish to change.

CUE EXPOSURE

The client is exposed to the temptation, with the goal of acquiring different methods of coping with the resultant impulsive urges. For example, a binge eater may sit in front of a plate of favourite food and attempt to resist the urge to eat it. Eventually, the urge subsides. The technique should first be used in a session enabling the wellness coach to help the client to develop coping strategies to deal with the cue. It is useful for the client in the session to rate, on a scale of 0 to 10, the strength of the urge. In the example given, coping strategies could include cognitive distraction, aversive therapy, coping statement and relaxation techniques.

HABIT CONTROL

Habit control interventions are designed to reduce or stop undesired habits, such as hair pulling, nail biting, stuttering or tics. For example, a client who pulls or twists her hair would be asked to clench her fists when she had an urge to pull.

MODELLING

Before a client undertakes an agreed-upon task, the coach demonstrates the desired behaviour in small, manageable steps. It is recommended that the coach emulate the client by demonstrating the particular skill at an acceptable standard and not in a 'perfect' manner. The client can practise the behaviour, such as communication skills within the session, as the wellness coach provides constructive feedback. The client is then assigned to demonstrate the skills in real life and report back on progress.

RESPONSE COST

This intervention is a method of self-control training in which clients agree to a penalty if they do not undertake a particular behaviour; for example, a client who wishes to stop smoking agrees to donate a sum of money to his least favourite political party if he smokes. It is useful if this intervention is paired with rewards, so that when the desired behaviour occurs the client rewards himself, for example by watching his favourite TV programme.

RESPONSE PREVENTION

This intervention is used with clients suffering from OCD. With this technique, clients are exposed to ritual-evoking cues or thoughts and they attempt to resist the urge to perform rituals. Wellness journals are used to monitor progress.

SELF-MONITORING AND RECORDING

Wellness journalling and daily logs are useful.

STIMULUS CONTROL

This method consists of changing the environment so that the client does not have easy access to the stimulus. For example, a client who wishes to stop smoking would remove cigarettes, ashtrays and matches from her home and would temporarily avoid visiting friends who smoked.

RELAXATION TECHNIQUES

Clients can be coached in progressive relaxation, breathing techniques or autogenic training. The physiological changes of these techniques can be monitored with biofeedback.

IMAGERY

When we get an internal 'picture', we are *visualizing* it. Think of your favourite food or holiday destination, and you'll see an image in your mind's eye. CBC imagery is using the power of the mind's eye to reframe a negative image into a more positive one. If your client is about to have a medical procedure, for example, he most likely 'sees' it negatively, pain and all. By using imagery, he can see a different picture, one where the procedure goes well and with less discomfort.

In order to identify images, evoke a faulty-thinking scenario. Ways of responding to a client's automatic image which accompanies faulty thinking include those detailed in Table 5.13.

Table 5.13 Imagery management techniques	
Jumping forward into the future	If the client keeps playing the 'Yes, but…' game, the technique of jumping forward one week, month or year to after the event can be useful.
Changing the ending of the image	This can be used with those suffering from PTSD. Instead of concluding on a negative note where the client is a victim, the client is helped to envisage a more positive and triumphant ending. The past cannot be changed and memories may be linked to real and negative life events (rather than thought distortions, e.g. catastrophizing). But clients can be trained to see themselves as now prepared, empowered and able to take control, should something similar happen again in the future.
Testing the image against objective reality	With this technique, the wellness coach treats the image like an automatic thought e.g. testing the validity.

Anti-future shock imagery	Palmer and Dryden (2005) ask clients to visualize themselves coping with future changes e.g. children leaving home. This technique can help deal with predicted life events and changes, e.g. surgery, death of someone close, retirement. Clients are asked to visualize themselves coping with different aspects of the future feared events. The technique can be used as a lapse reduction technique in the ending stage of wellness coaching to help clients cope with future unexpected problems.
Aversive imagery	Palmer and Dryden (2005) encourage clients to link undesirable behaviours, e.g. excessive eating or smoking, with unpleasant images. This helps clients to reduce or stop the frequency of times they undertake the undesirable response. For example, when clients on a smoking cessation programme are offered a cigarette and they immediately visualize tar accumulating in the lungs. This may reduce the likelihood of the cigarette being accepted. Another client on a weight-control programme can imagine someone he dislikes vomiting over the food he is about to eat. The client should choose the unpleasant image and use it for five minutes at a time.
Motivation imagery	This is a variation of time-projection imagery to help motivate clients to deal with their problems. Clients are asked to visualize their future based on avoiding their problems (inaction), including all the associated disadvantages. Then they are asked to contrast this picture with another view of their future based on dealing with their problems (action), including all the associated advantages. This technique is useful when clients are not prepared to face their fears. Inaction imagery must come before action imagery
Rational-emotive imagery	Palmer and Dryden (2005) guide clients to change their irrational beliefs about a disturbing situation while imaging the situation. Clients are instructed to imagine a feared situation and simultaneously repeat a previously negotiated coping statement to themselves. This helps clients experience less anxiety and to prepare for difficult situations. Rating the strength of the emotion before, during and after exercise helps the wellness coach to assess the appropriateness of the chosen coping statement.

Table 5.13 Imagery management techniques *cont.*	
Time-projection imagery	This technique guides a client backward or forward in time to relive past events or to see that a present negative event has been overcome in the future.
Associated imagery	Palmer and Dryden (2005) guide clients to discover sources of negative emotions that appear to come from nowhere. Clients are guided to focus on and increase the negative feelings and to see what images enter their minds.
Implosion	Palmer and Dryden (2005) ask clients to imagine prolonged exposure to their most feared situation until their anxiety subsides or they get used to it. This is used with clients who could deal with a high exposure to anxiety. A similar technique is imagined exposure where a hierarchy of fears is used. Clients rate these fears on a scale of 1 to 10 and then work their way through these fears until they feel comfortable.
Step-up technique	Palmer and Dryden (2005) ask clients to picture various outcomes of a feared situation leading or approaching the worst possible outcome and then cope with or survive that situation. This can be used if a client is anxious about a probable future event such as surgery, and her underlying beliefs have been difficult to determine. The client is instructed to imagine the feared situation unfolding. It might be useful to ask the client to 'step up' the scene by visualizing the very worst possible outcome. Then the client and wellness coach consider how the situation could be dealt with, and subsequently the client is asked to repeat the exercise incorporating the new coping strategies.
Time-tripping	Palmer and Dryden (2005) count with the client either forward or backward in time, with aim of the client healing past situations or seeing himself in a positive situation in the future.
Trauma-coping imagery	Palmer and Dryden (2005) help clients experiencing a traumatic event to find an alternative, more positive 'ending' that can be used if they experience flashbacks or obsessive thoughts.

BIBLIOTHERAPY

This consists of clients using relevant self-help manuals and books. Leaflets, audio material, DVDs and CDs at the wellness coach's suggestion may help clients understand the nature of their particular problem.

COLLAPSED-COPING STATEMENT

Once clients have developed a coping statement, they are more prepared to confront their issues. However, long-winded coping statements can be difficult to remember under pressure. Therefore, helpful beliefs need to be shortened or 'collapsed' into one or two words that have personal meaning for clients and are easy to recall.

DE-CATASTROPHIZING CONTINUUM

When clients are overestimating the negative outcome of events, they are making thinking errors such as magnification and all-or-nothing thinking. De-catastrophizing demonstrates to clients that bad things are seldom the end of the world. By using a 'continuum of badness' scale from 1 to 10, the wellness coach asks the client to state how bad the situation will be. After practising wellness tasks, the client is asked again to use the continuum.

DESERTED-ISLAND TECHNIQUE

This technique demonstrates that holding on to unhelpful beliefs and not necessarily the activating event can lead to a heightened emotional disturbance and trigger emotions such as anger, guilt, anxiety or depression.

LETTER-WRITING

A useful between-session activity is to ask clients to write a letter to the person with whom they have issues, but they don't send it.

THOUGHT-STOPPING

The client is asked to think about the obsessive thought or image. Once the client has invoked it, he is coached in performing a distraction activity, such as clapping, shouting 'Stop!', pinging an elastic band or scrunchie round his wrist, or imagining a road stop sign or a red traffic light.

BEHAVIOURAL EXPERIMENTS

The wellness coach and client look ahead at the probable consequences to give the best conditions for success to be achieved (in relation to agreed assignments between sessions) and pay attention to practical difficulties or faulty thinking which may prevent the assignment from being carried out. It is important to convey to the client that this is an experiment and that carrying it out is success in itself, irrespective of the outcome. The aim is to elicit some response which contraindicates or fails to support a particular thought or belief.

COMPARING SELF WITH OTHERS

This can be useful to aid distancing and separating the client from the pattern of regarding herself as the focal point of all events. The wellness coach asks the client to think of others who do not hold the client's unhelpful beliefs but whom she regards favourably, or do hold the client's unhelpful beliefs (to her detriment). The coach will ask the client to select another who has similar or opposite beliefs, depending upon the aim of the particular intervention; a mentor or role model might be chosen. The client can then consider the effect of adopting the more helpful beliefs she assumes the mentor to have. She is led to recognize that another does not hold her belief yet functions more effectively. By comparison, the client recognizes that she can modify her own beliefs without adverse consequences and with probable benefits. An opposite approach is to select another who does hold the unhelpful belief but suffers as a consequence. It is often easier for clients to generate meaningful and believable counters to others' unhelpful beliefs than to their own. This enables distance from the unhelpful belief to be achieved.

Reduction of distress (or referral)

As you go through the process of exploring and challenging faulty thinking, the client will ideally experience a change in mindset, reduction in emotional distress and a positive change in behaviour. If this continually doesn't seem to be happening and if the client doesn't engage with negotiated tasks, it might be that the client is not coaching-ready or needs referral to a clinical therapist.

Let's see how we might facilitate Tom's journey when it comes to exploring and challenging faulty thinking with regard to his goals.

FINDING WAYS TO LESSEN WORK INTERRUPTIONS
(Phone calls to be diverted to secretary; work two days a week from home)

Identifying faulty thinking:

- It's going to be impossible to find ways to lessen work interruptions.
- My secretary has got too much on her plate to take any more tasks on.
- Will I be disciplined enough to work from home?
- They'll just chase me up at home – there's no getting away from them!

Consequences of staying with faulty thinking:

- I'll carry on getting work interruptions which will delay my getting work done. I'll continue feel drained and resentful because I'll spend too much time on work and not enough with family.

Self-disputing process:

- I know there are ways to lessen work interruptions.

- I assume my secretary has got too much on her plate. I'm sure she can take this task on if she organizes it properly.

- I have worked from home before and it has worked out well.

- People won't phone me up at home. All calls will be diverted to my secretary.

Effective reduction of distress:

- Increased effectiveness of completing work. More family time. I feel more relaxed.

DELEGATING TASKS

(Bert to do the monthly spreadsheets; retail emails could have a separate email address and Anna could check them to filter out important ones)

Identifying faulty thinking:

- Can Bert cope with the spreadsheets?

- Bert will think I'm a nuisance.

- I need to organize a new email address with IT. Can I be bothered?

- How will Anna know the important emails to filter through?

- I must do everything (belief).

Consequences of staying with faulty thinking:

- I'll be doing tasks that aren't necessary for me to do. I'll continue feel drained and resentful because I'm spending too much time on work and not enough with family.

Self-disputing process:

- I'm going to speak with Bert to see if he needs further training on spreadsheets.

- I'm mind-reading what Bert will think. He might not be overjoyed at the extra work. On the other hand, he might welcome the opportunity.

- Once the new email address has been set up with IT, another task will be done and less work for me.
- Anna will know the important emails to filter through because I will give her a list.
- It's OK not to do everything. I am still a competent manager.

Effective reduction of distress:

- Increased effectiveness of completing work. More family time. I feel more relaxed.

TIME MANAGEMENT
(Filter non-important meetings; find alternative ways of attending others, e.g. tele-conferencing)

Identifying faulty thinking:

- There are so many meetings, how can I organize this?
- I'll have to contact so many people.
- I wish someone else would think of organizing meetings in another way – why does it have to be me who initiates these things?

Consequences of staying with faulty thinking:

- I'll be attending meetings when I don't really need to. I'll continue feeling drained and resentful because I'm spending too much time on work and not enough with family.

Self-disputing process:

- I attend around 12 meetings a month. I need to identify optional ways of contributing and gaining meeting outcomes.
- My secretary can contact key personnel with alternatives and filter responses back to me.
- Maybe other attendees feel similar to myself. I've got the initiative to do something about it.

Effective reduction of distress:

- Increased effectiveness of completing work. More family time. I feel more relaxed.

TALKING TO BOSS
Identifying faulty thinking:

- She'll never listen to me.
- What can she do to help me?
- She'll think I'm feeble.
- I must always be in control (belief).

Consequences of staying with faulty thinking:

- I'll be angry at my boss. I'll continue feel drained and resentful because I'm spending too much time on work and not enough with family.

Self-disputing process:

- Mary has always listened before and had some good observations. She probably doesn't know how stretched I am.
- Mary may come up with some good ideas I haven't thought of to make my life easier.
- I know from our feedback sessions that Mary values my contribution. She has a record for being fair to her team.
- I am in control by choosing to talk with my boss.

Effective reduction of distress:

- Increased effectiveness of completing work. More family time. I feel more relaxed.

Step 6: Decision-making and action planning

Self-monitoring through assignments serves several functions. By setting between-session assignments, clients can objectively test out new ways of thinking and behaving, and the results can provide new information to themselves and the wellness coach. Self-monitoring puts responsibility into the hands of clients and can be used as a baseline for assessing or measuring behavioural change and improvement.

The goal has been set, faulty thinking and beliefs reframed and choices made. Now decisions need to occur. Use this seven-step process to help clients:

- Gather information to make a list of choices.
- Consider the pros and cons for each choice.
- Rate each choice by importance from 1 to 10.
- Consider any beliefs or fears affecting their thinking.

- Project themselves six months or a year into the future and then look backwards at the decision they made. Decide which decision looks best from there.

- Make the decision.

- Evaluate their decision. If clients don't like how things are progressing, they can do something else.

Negotiating wellness tasks with clients

Wellness tasks reinforce and consolidate learning and confirm the client's commitment to work towards his chosen goal. He is more likely to complete assignments or engage in activities he would rather avoid if these are scheduled as part of the session. In order to increase the likelihood of completing wellness tasks, the following is suggested:

- Wellness tasks should be uncomplicated and specific. The client should understand what he has agreed to do and the reasons for choosing those particular tasks. The coach should check for any uncertainty that would hinder the client's ability to complete the task.

- It is important that wellness tasks are formulated, discussed and agreed collaboratively.

- Where underlying beliefs are being challenged, assignments should be completed a number of times to reinforce the learning.

- Before embarking on a task, the coach should test the client's commitment to carry out the work and explore resistance, or negotiate a more appealing task.

- Tailor the assignment to the client.

- Often a task feels overwhelming and the client fears he will not cope. To make the task more manageable, the client and coach can breakdown goals into achievable chunks.

- Facilitate ways the client can remember to do the assignment.

- Anticipate possible problems and discuss possible solutions.

- Prepare for a possible negative outcome.

Tom's decisions are:

- to speak with secretary and divert phone calls

- to set up working from home two days a week and to divert calls to secretary

- to speak with Bert about taking the spreadsheet task on and ask if he needs further training
- to set up the new email address with IT
- to speak with Anna about filtering through important emails and to provide her with a priority list
- to identify optional ways of contributing and gaining meeting outcomes for the identified meetings
- for secretary to contact key personnel and to filter responses to me
- for secretary to set up a meeting with Mary so we can talk things through.

Step 7: Implementation

The goals have been set and decisions made. Now the client implements action.

Managing progress and accountability

Although clients are ultimately responsible for their decisions and actions, as their wellness coach you have the ability to hold attention on what is important for them while leaving responsibility with them to take action. Your role at the stage of implementation is to:

- negotiate actions with the client that will move her towards her stated goals
- demonstrate follow-through by asking the client about those actions that she committed to during the previous session
- acknowledge the client for what she has done, not done, learned or become aware of since the previous session
- keep the client on track between sessions by focusing on the wellness coaching plan and outcomes, while being open to adjusting behaviours and actions based on the client's processes
- facilitate the small steps while being mindful of the bigger picture of where the client wishes to go
- promote the client's self-discipline, and hold the client accountable for what she says she is going to do and for the results of an intended action
- develop the client's ability to make decisions, address key concerns, develop herself, determine priorities, set the pace of learning, and reflect on and learn from experiences
- confront the client constructively when she does not take agreed-upon actions.

Correcting and improving the performance of a client by way of constructive confrontation is one of the basic responsibilities of the wellness coach at the implementation stage. By knowing the attitudes and personality traits of your client, you can provide feedback in a constructive way. Be sure your own attitude is one of genuine helpfulness when criticizing. If a performance seems to be lacking, get all the facts first. Bad performance might be due to factors beyond the control of the client. Clients respond much better if they believe that their wellness coach has faith in them and thinks they have the ability and intelligence to do the task correctly. Don't belittle clients. Personal abuse wounds the ego to the extent it's not possible to listen with an open mind. On the other hand, constructive suggestions will motivate clients to improve. If there is a performance issue, show the way to eliminate it and how to substitute the right action. Explain how and why the task needs to be done in the manner expected.

Step 8: Evaluation

Implementation has occurred. The client now needs to evaluate the process and outcome and to consider how it worked for him and what he might like or need to change.

Tom's overall goal was to not bring work home, therefore having more quality time with family. We now need to evaluate Tom's performance (behaviour) outcome. Tom needs to do this, and you need to contribute. Monitor the process and outcome for each goal. Consider all the factors that affect the achievement of goals, whether positive or negative. Assess how the client achieved a specific milestone in the path towards achieving a particular wellness goal (this will make the next milestones easier to reach). If a certain goal was not achieved or was achieved unsatisfactorily, explore what went wrong so that the client does not repeat the same mistake again. Re-evaluate goals where appropriate to make them more challenging if they were reached easily, or make them easier in case of difficulty in achievement. Measure the client's personal growth and development in relation to wellness. What wellness-related mindsets have changed and how?

CPD task sheet

This is your Continuing Professional Development (CPD) task sheet which summarizes key module points and offers you the opportunity to engage with tasks to deepen your learning.

Module summary

- Cognitive behavioural coaching skills need to be woven throughout your wellness coaching sessions and will help your client identify problems, explore choices and consequences, select goals, explore and challenge faulty thinking, make decisions, action plan, implement change and evaluate outcomes.

Your tasks

1. Follow the eight steps with a process of your own.
2. Follow the eight steps through with an existing client you know well.

Module 6
Additional Skills for Wellness Coaching

By the end of this module, you will have explored some of the additional skills useful for wellness coaching which might also serve as CPD options.

You are already a qualified therapist in your own field, and I wouldn't presume to tell you how to work on your CPD in relation to that area. However, a range of additional wellness coaching skills might be useful to you, and you may consider taking further training in or a course of informal study.

Biofeedback

With biofeedback, clients are trained to control certain bodily processes that normally occur involuntarily such as heart rate, muscle activity, skin temperature, skin resistance, brain surface electrical activity and blood pressure. These processes are measured and displayed on a monitor. The client is first coached in relaxation skills which are practised regularly. With the help of wellness coaching, clients can use then gauge their body's reaction to regular relaxation via biofeedback to lessen the effects of conditions such as pain, stress, insomnia and headaches.

Three professional biofeedback organizations – the Association for Applied Psychophysiology and Biofeedback, Biofeedback Certification Institution of America, and the International Society for Neurofeedback and Research – arrived at a consensus definition of biofeedback in 2008:

> Biofeedback is a process that enables an individual to learn how to change physiological activity for the purposes of improving health and performance. Precise instruments measure physiological activity such as brainwaves, heart function, breathing, muscle activity, and skin temperature. These instruments rapidly and accurately 'feed back' information to the user. The presentation of this information – often in conjunction with changes in thinking, emotions, and behaviour

– supports desired physiological changes. Over time, these changes can endure without continued use of an instrument. (Association for Applied Psychophysiology and Biofeedback 2008)

> ### Inside tip
>
> If you are using biofeedback as part of a workshop, participants usually love to have a go. Be mindful that if you demonstrate the equipment, you are likely to experience performance stress!

Stress management

Stress is a generic word used to describe our response to a life event. Our coping strategies determine how we respond to acute or chronic stress. What may be deemed *stressful* by one person may not be by another. It is possible for this response to reach a threshold of distress which causes physical or psychological symptoms and a reduction in function. At these times, clients need to be coached in stress-management techniques, which may include relaxation coaching, meditation or cognitive behavioural coaching. These techniques help to get the client back in control and develop stress resilience. While there are a number of stress-management courses which offer CPD and qualification opportunities, it may also be worthwhile to consider the different aspects of stress management and doing more focused training in each area.

> ### Inside tip
>
> Stress-management coaching is a biggie and can be transferred across a plethora of wellness needs. I've worked with individuals on work-related stress, exam stress, presentation anxiety and stress linked to progressive and terminal illnesses.

Cognitive behavioural coaching (CBC)

We have briefly covered this approach in Module 5. However, as you are likely to be using CBC extensively in wellness coaching, I suggest you do further training.

> ### Inside tip
>
> Once you have a good foundation in CBC, you can specialize in, for example, low self-esteem, social anxiety and shyness, chronic pain, anger, depression, anxiety, chronic fatigue, insomnia, chronic medical problems, weight problems or body image.

Relaxation techniques

Relaxation techniques are designed to relieve tension. Specific techniques may be aimed at lowering blood pressure or easing muscle tension and can be used with other techniques such as meditation, guided imagery or hypnotherapy. There are three major types of relaxation techniques:

Autogenic training (AT)

AT was developed in the early years of the 20th century by the psychiatrist and neurologist Dr Johannes Schultz (Luthe and Schultz 1969). During the core of AT, clients learn a series of mental exercises allowing them to enter deep states of relaxation. The exercises consist of the silent repetition of simple formulae while focusing on bodily sensations that are associated with relaxation: warmth and heaviness in the limbs, warmth in the solar plexus, regularity of heartbeat, etc. An essential feature of AT is that the exercises are carried out in a state of passive concentration with the client observing all that happens but unconcerned with achievement. In this state, natural self-regulatory mechanisms are able to function optimally, leading to a rebalancing of activity between the left and right brain hemispheres. According to the British Autogenic Society (2007), there are:

- clinical applications for general problems, e.g. insomnia and free-floating anxiety, migraine, arthritis, colitis, IBS and high blood pressure

- non-clinical applications which appear to rebalance our mental faculties and bring closer harmony between the analytical left hemisphere of the brain and the more emotional, inspirational and creative right hemisphere.

Progressive muscle relaxation (PMR)

One of the simplest techniques for relaxation is PMR, a widely-used procedure that was developed by Jacobson in 1938. The PMR procedure teaches clients to relax their muscles through a two-step process. First, the client deliberately applies tension to certain muscle groups, and then stops the tension and turns his attention to noticing how the muscles relax as the tension flows away. Through repetitive practice, he learns to recognize and distinguish the difference between a tensed muscle and a completely relaxed muscle. With this knowledge, he can induce physical muscular relaxation at the first signs of the tension or anxiety.

Breathing techniques

When we are tense, we tend to breathe shallowly. Bad breathing causes light headedness, hyperventilation, headaches and makes stress worse. Breathing techniques, such as slowdown breathing, abdominal breathing, square breathing, countdown breathing and alternate nose breathing can help clients to regain control of the breath.

Inside tip

Another must-do piece of training: because so many wellness issues are stress-related or anxiety-ridden, coaching the client to physically relax is crucial.

Humanistic psychology

Humanistic psychology began in the 1950s and includes such movers and shakers as Abraham Maslow and Carl Rogers. According to the Association of Humanistic Psychology Practitioners (2010), the fundamental core beliefs are:

> The individual is unique, while being part of the environment, including relationships with others within the larger systems of humankind, incorporating family, community and society, and with the natural world. The individual is neither intrinsically good nor bad and is motivated toward self actualization and to seek security, love, belonging and, ultimately, truth. A person is greater than the sum of their parts, which includes their body, behaviours, beliefs (secular and spiritual), thoughts and feelings (conscious and unconscious). The person is an integrated and self regulating whole, only when this balance is disturbed or incomplete do dis-ease and dysfunction arise as symptoms, rather than as causes. Accordingly individuals have a right to autonomy and self determination, subject to accepting responsibility for their own actions. Each individual also has responsibility toward others, respecting their rights and honouring difference and diversity.

> ### Inside tip
>
> Humanistic psychology is a non-directive approach, therefore knowing more about the theory and techniques would be useful to wellness coaching.

Flower remedies

Flower essences have been used for centuries in Australia, South America, Asia, Egypt, South America and India. Now, there is a growing movement towards realignment with nature, and flower essences are among those ancient steps re-emerging as part of integrated healthcare. Flower essences utilize the essence's positive energy to transmute a negative state. Each flower conveys a subtle energy pattern which is transferred to water during essence preparation. This preparation is then used in various ways internally or externally. Flower essences treat personality characteristics, rather than the physical complaints, in order to rebalance the psycho-emotional self so that the life force can become the healer. The belief that we can heal ourselves is the basis of flower-essence philosophy. Flower essences do not directly treat the physical body or its symptoms. From a spiritual perspective, they address mental and emotional imbalances that, if left unresolved, could influence the wellness of the physical body. Essences do not affect us biochemically as does traditional allopathic medicine. They are water-based products that have no chemical or biological materials present other than the water and a preservative such as brandy or vodka.

> ### Inside tip
>
> I don't use flower remedies with every wellness coaching client. Sometimes clients ask me if I use them and other times, when it seems appropriate, I offer to make up a remedy. If flower remedies appeal to you, I recommend you explore the Bach Flower Remedies and the Australian Bush Flower Essences.

Visualization and imagery

Visualization is using the mind's eye to visualize a relaxing scene or the positive outcome of a difficult medical procedure. The visualization is normally representational – that is, we recognize what we see.

Imagery is using the power of the mind in a more abstract way. This technique is often used in pain management or to help the mind heal the body, such as IBS or cancer. Imagery is very individually driven. The client comes up with the images. When another person takes a client through the visualization or imagery process (a wellness coach or CD, for example), it is called guided visualization or guided imagery. Both of these techniques should be part of the wellness coach's toolbox and can be used with great effect.

Inside tip

I use imagery and visualization a lot in my wellness coaching work. Some examples of when I have used these techniques with clients include nurses preparing patients for surgery, preparing cancer patients for chemotherapy, soothing IBS symptoms, mental health nurses working with patients, public speaking, managing migraines and improving relationships.

Nutrition

Nutrition can play a big part in the wellness coaching process. If you are already a qualified nutritional therapist, you are well placed to extend your coaching services. If you are considering developing your skills in this area, you may be interested in the definition of a nutritional therapist as opposed to a dietician or nutritionist:

> For nutritional therapists (who practise complementary and alternative medicine) optimum nutrition encompasses individual prescriptions for diet and lifestyle in order to alleviate or prevent ailments and to promote optimal gene expression through all life stages. Recommendations may include guidance on natural detoxification, procedures to promote colon health, methods to support digestion and absorption, the avoidance of toxins or allergens and the appropriate use of supplementary nutrients, including phytonutrients. Nutritional therapists advise on each person's unique dietary and nutritional needs for metabolic and hormonal homeostasis, using a variety of biochemical and functional tests to inform recommended protocols and programmes. (British Association for Applied Nutrition and Nutritional Therapy 2011)

> **Inside tip**
>
> I specialize in coaching clients with specific conditions and often this includes nutrition.

Communication skills

This vast area covers assertiveness, public speaking and presentation skills, anger management, negotiation skills, conflict management and interpersonal communication. Not every wellness issue has a physical label on it. Many are communication related; for example, I've worked with several men on anger management (and a few women, too, with the extra label of *PMT* on it). Work-related stress issues are often linked to an inappropriate communication style.

> **Inside tip**
>
> Wellness coaching involving communication skills is popular. For example, relationship coaching covers areas such as survival after divorce, dating, intimacy and relationship stress. As well as one-to-one coaching and group coaching, you could offer couples coaching.

Meditation

Meditation refers to a group of techniques including transcendental meditation, mindfulness, mantra meditation and Zen Buddhist meditation. Most techniques started in Eastern religious or spiritual traditions and have been used by different cultures throughout the world for thousands of years. Today many people use meditation outside of its traditional religious or cultural settings, for wellness. The practice can result in increased calmness, physical relaxation and psychological balance.

> A 2007 national Government survey that asked about CAM use in a sample of 23,393 U.S. adults found that 9.4 percent of respondents (representing more than 20 million people) had used meditation in the past 12 months—compared with 7.6 percent of respondents (representing more than 15 million people) in a similar survey conducted in 2002. The 2007 survey also asked about CAM use in a sample of 9,417 children; 1 percent (representing 725,000 children)

had used meditation in the past 12 months. (National Center for Complementary and Alternative Medicine 2010)

People use meditation for various health problems such as anxiety, pain, depression, stress, insomnia and physical or emotional symptoms associated with chronic illnesses and their treatment such as heart disease, HIV/AIDS and cancer. Meditation is also used for overall wellness.

> ### Inside tip
>
> In my experience, many clients have preconceived idea of meditation – normally one of sitting cross-legged for hours and humming tunelessly. There are a huge range of practical and simple meditations to help relax the body and focus the mind.

Reiki

Everything, including our body, is energy (Japanese call it *ki*, Chinese call it *chi* or *qi*, Indians call it *prana*) in various states of vibration and motion. Healing practitioners work with this energy to promote healing and Reiki (pronounced *ray-key*) is one way of channelling this energy. Reiki is a generic word in Japan, and is used to describe many types of healing and spiritual work. Reiki can be useful in wellness coaching, especially if you are a Reiki II practitioner, which deals with the emotional and mental levels of well-being.

> ### Inside tip
>
> As a Reiki teacher, I use this method in a number of ways with wellness coaching clients. I always use it to help balance the mental and emotional energy of the client. No hands-on treatment is required; just the compassionate setting of intent as the session starts. For clients who are keen on Reiki, I may offer them a hands-on Reiki session to start with, as this opens them up wonderfully. Sometimes I might offer it as a 15-minute end to the session.

Pain management

Pain management is the control of pain or discomfort through medication, stress reduction, relaxation, biofeedback, exercise, cognitive behavioural coaching, massage or hydrotherapy. As well as studying the physiology and psychology of pain, it is a good idea to learn more about the specific techniques which manage pain.

Inside tip

I tend to use pain management with pregnancy coaching more than anything.

Gestalt

Gestalt therapy was developed by Fritz and Laura Perls and Paul Goodman in the 1940s (Perls, Hefferline and Goodman 1951). It is a form of psychotherapy that emphasizes personal responsibility and focuses upon the individual's experience in the present moment, the therapist/coach–client relationship, the environmental and social contexts of a person's life, and the self-regulating adjustments a person makes as a result of her overall situation.

Inside tip

Gestalt is not something I use a great deal in my wellness coaching practice – but my supervisor has used it with me!

Emotional intelligence

'Emotional intelligence' refers to the ability to perceive, control and evaluate emotions. Since 1990, Peter Salovey and John D. Mayer have been the leading researchers on emotional intelligence. In their article *Emotional Intelligence*, they defined emotional intelligence as 'the subset of social intelligence that involves the ability to monitor one's own and others' feelings and emotions, to discriminate among them and to use this information to guide one's thinking and actions' (Salovey and Mayer 1990).

Inside tip

CBC utilizes many emotional intelligence techniques.

Transactional analysis (TA)

TA is a theory of personality and human interaction developed by Dr Eric Berne in the late 1950s. According to the International Transactional Analysis Association, 'TA is a theory of personality and a systematic psychotherapy for personal growth and personal change' (Stewart and Joines 1987, p.3). As a theory of personality, TA describes how people are structured psychologically and uses the ego-state (parent–child–adult) model to do this. This model helps explain how people function and express their personality in their behaviour.

Inside tip

TA is another technique I often use in wellness coaching especially when relationships are involved. I use TA in two ways. One is to help clients make sense of the parent, child and adult and how they relate to each other within themselves. Second, I help clients understand how these parts of them relate to those parts in another.

Solution-focused brief therapy

The solution-focused approach was developed in America in the 1980s by Steve de Shazer and Insoo Kim Berg. It is based on solution-building rather than problem-solving and explores current resources and future hopes rather than present problems and past causes (Institute for Solution-Focused Therapy 2010).

Rational emotive behaviour therapy (REBT)

REBT created and developed by Albert Ellis, psychotherapist and psychologist, who holds that humans are prone to adopting irrational beliefs and behaviours which stand in the way of their achieving their goals (Neenan and Dryden 1999). Often, these irrational attitudes take the form of 'should' and 'must' and conflict with rational desires and preferences. REBT focuses on uncovering irrational beliefs which may lead to unhealthy negative emotions and replacing them with more productive rational alternatives.

Inside tip

Yet another CBC approach. You can read more about this approach in Module 5.

Environmental wellness

Practitioners of environmental medicine recognize that illness can be caused by a broad range of substances, including chemicals found at home, in the workplace, and in the air, water and food. There are multiple approaches to treatment including changes in lifestyle, diet and environment. Studies have supported the use of the approaches of environmental medicine in treating arthritis, asthma, chemical sensitivity, allergies, colitis, depression, eczema, fatigue and hyperactivity.

According to the British Society for Ecological Medicine (2009), 'Ecological medicine addresses the interactions between the individual and the environment and their health consequences – both the impact of environmental factors on the individual, and that of each individual's actions on the environment, upon which we all depend'. There are five interlacing aspects: nutrition, toxins (pollutants and environmental toxins), allergy, individuality (inherited and acquired individuality determines our ability to cope with altered states of nutrition and toxicity, and with multiple other stresses) and environment.

Inside tip

Environmental medicine is a key part of wellness coaching and needs to be part of your toolbox.

Medical qigong

Medical qigong (pronounced *chee-GUNG*) is a component of traditional Chinese medicine that combines movement, meditation and regulation of breathing to enhance the flow of *qi* (vital energy) in order to maintain health and heal disease. It is believed that the regular practice of medical qigong helps to cleanse the body of toxins, restore energy, reduce anxiety and stress, and help individuals maintain a healthy and active lifestyle.

Medical qigong treatment has been officially recognized as a standard medical technique in Chinese hospitals since 1989. China began officially managing qigong through government regulation in 1996 and listed qigong as part of their national health plan.

> ### Inside tip
>
> I have experienced qigong and have an image of qigong wellness in my coaching room on the information board. The process isn't for everyone, but medical qigong in particular can be quite profound.

Journalling

Wellness journalling offers a private place for stress reduction, healing, personal growth, self-awareness and problem-solving.

> ### Inside tip
>
> I used journaling when I went through my breast cancer journey and have used it several times since to work through difficult issues. Not all clients like this approach, but it's always worth running past them. It's like the client has a silent wellness coach or therapist they can relate to 24/7.

Emotional Freedom Technique (EFT)

EFT is a self-help mechanism based on the discovery that imbalances in the body's energy system have profound effects on one's personal psychology. Correcting these imbalances, which is done by tapping on certain body locations, often leads to rapid recoveries (Craig undated).

> ### Inside tip
>
> I don't use EFT myself, but I have several wellness colleagues who swear by it.

Positive psychology

Positive psychology is a science of positive aspects of human life, such as happiness and well-being. It is a recent branch of psychology (with roots in humanistic psychology) whose purpose was summed up by psychologists Martin Seligman and Mihaly Csikszentmihalyi (2000): 'We believe that a psychology of positive human functioning will arise that achieves a scientific understanding and effective interventions to build thriving in individuals, families, and communities' (p.9).

Inside tip

Positive psychology is a fantastic approach as long as it isn't used as a psychological sticking plaster.

Neuro-Linguistic Programming (NLP)

NLP was developed as a therapy in the 1970s by linguist John Grinder and Dr Richard Bandler, an information scientist with specific interest in understanding cognitive brain-based thinking patterns (Tosey and Mathison 2006). At NLP's core is a wide range of methods and models that aim to create an understanding of thought processes, behaviour and change management. To break down the title looks something like this:

Neuro refers to how the mind processes through the senses, e.g. sounds, tastes, tactile awareness, smells, internal images and sensations.

Linguistic refers to how the information is received by attributing language to the sounds, tastes, tactile awareness, smells, internal images and sensations which form our daily awareness.

Programming refers to the behavioural patterns or 'programmes' that occur as a result of the neurological filtering and linguistic processes.

NLP techniques are useful when wanting to generate creativity, making changes for personal and professional achievement, improving performance and increasing confidence.

Inside tip

NLP is widely used in the coaching industry. I find similarity between NLP and CBC.

Multimodal therapy (MMT)

Arnold Lazarus, a behaviour therapist, developed MMT (Palmer 2010). This eclectic and psycho-educational approach would fit into a cognitive behaviour form of coaching which attends all modalities of human functioning and is presented in the acronym **BASICID** as:

- **B:** Behaviour
- **A:** Affect (emotions)
- **S:** Sensation (touch, smell, sight, hearing, taste)
- **I:** Imagery (thinking in pictures, self-image)
- **C:** Cognition (thinking in words, beliefs, attitudes, opinions, thinking styles)
- **I:** Interpersonal (how we relate to others)
- **D:** Drugs and biology (medications, substances, diet, exercise, general health, sleep)

The client presents with a wellness issue, for example IBS. The BASICID blueprint is used as a basic assessment from which each modality is explored in relation to the wellness issue. For example, how do you behave when the IBS is at its worst? What cognition do you have of the IBS when it is griping your stomach? From this point, different techniques can be used to work with each modality addressing the wellness issue. For example, for the behaviour modality, behaviour rehearsal may be appropriate. For the cognition modality, constructive self-talk may be appropriate.

Inside tip

I use multimodal approaches with stress coaching more than any other issue.

Mindfulness-based stress reduction (MBSR)

Dr Jon Kabat-Zinn developed MBSR programme at the University of Massachusetts Medical Centre in 1979 (Mindful Living Programs 2010). MBSR incorporates techniques such as meditation, gentle yoga and mindbody exercises. Since its inception, MBSR has evolved into a common form of complementary medicine with an additional curative role in a variety of health problems including stress, asthma, high blood pressure, chronic pain and insomnia. It is also used as a preventative aid for health enhancement.

> ### Inside tip
>
> When one of my cats went missing for five days, I practised mindfulness and it really helped me (the cat returned unharmed). It is a difficult art to master and you need to practise yourself before working with others.

CPD task sheet

This is your Continuing Professional Development (CPD) task sheet which summarizes key module points and offers you the opportunity to engage with tasks to deepen your learning.

Module summary

- Biofeedback, stress management, cognitive behavioural coaching, relaxation techniques, humanistic psychology, flower remedies, visualization and imagery, nutrition, communication skills, meditation, Reiki, pain management, Gestalt, emotional intelligence, transactional analysis, solution-focused brief therapy, rational emotive behaviour therapy, environmental medicine, medical qigong, journalling, emotional freedom technique, positive psychology, neuro-linguistic programming, multimodal therapy and mindfulness-based stress reduction are all valuable bolt-ons to wellness coaching.

Your task

Identify two techniques from the above list and research them further including training options.

Applying Wellness Coaching

Part 3 lays out how you can apply an integrated therapeutic coaching approach to specific wellness niches. It assumes therapists have specific discipline-related skills and knowledge and will include these in their wellness coaching practice.

Module 7: Niching Wellness Coaching

Module 8: Applying Wellness Coaching

Module 9: Marketing Wellness Coaching

Module 7
Niching Wellness Coaching

By the end of the module, you will have explored:

- Choosing a niche market
- Niche market ideas
- Creating a diverse business model
- Your five-step plan to finding your wellness coaching niche

Choosing a niche market

You understand the basic knowledge and skills required for wellness coaching. Now let's talk business.

Being a generalist in reflexology or homeopathy puts you in the same category as the other 40 reflexologists and homeopaths in your area. Specializing in IBS or cancer care puts you in a different category. Working with children with IBS or cancer niches you down even more. It makes you stand out because you are addressing problems to which people can relate. You are niching your services.

In order to create a popular and profitable wellness coaching practice, you need to position and market your wellness coaching business to a specific group or niche market. When you address his challenges and show you can deliver solutions, your wellness coaching shopper is a step nearer to being a buyer. By being unique and focused on a core market, you can become an expert. People have more faith in you; therefore they are more likely to buy.

Whether you're doing wellness coaching with the CEO of a major company, a pregnant woman, or an athlete, you are coaching her about her wellness. But if you try to market the notion of wellness coaching to all three (who have very different needs), you'll spend a lot of time marketing and little time coaching. In other words, staying a generalist means working very hard for little money. So, do you want to offer executive wellness, pregnancy coaching or performance wellness?

It's not what you sell that matters, it's to whom. Look for clear, targetable markets with easily identifiable needs or problems, and consider whether you can fill their need or solve their problem. In order to achieve this, you need to do market research.

What is a niche?

A niche is a cross-section between a targeted segmentation of a particular market and your speciality. For example:

Your overall market: Teacher wellness.

Your market segment: Secondary-school teachers.

Your niche speciality: Coaching new secondary school teachers to manage their stress levels.

A viable niche market is well defined and accessible (you should be able to find them in groups). It has identifiable needs and desires with the disposable income to invest in coaching. Niche markets are a group that you have inside knowledge about – which usually means you're either a part of that group now or once were.

Reasons why you should choose a niche market

Finding and developing wellness coaching niches takes time and effort. The benefits of niching to you are to:

- build visibility and credibility faster
- reduce competition
- create a distinctive brand for your coaching business
- command higher fees (niche specialists can charge more)
- network with the movers and shakers in your market
- make your marketing more targeted saving time and money
- become an integral part of the industry
- gain in-depth knowledge and understanding of client challenges
- improve your skills
- increase your confidence
- build kudos.

With all the competition vying for your market's attention, it's almost impossible to be better than the competition. Your goal is to be different, not better. Separate yourself from your competitors. Small businesses try to be all things to all people in order to generate more sales, but the more general you are, the more indifferent you will appear to your audience. Specialization generates the perception of expertise. For example, a counsellor specializing in relationship issues will acquire more clients than a general counsellor might. By finding, filling and dominating a niche, you can become an expert.

Inside tip

Look to your skills set for niche ideas. Do you have a talent, passion or track record that could evolve into a wellness coaching niche?

Research the trends

When you think you've identified a skills set you would like to use and develop, look at the market forces and see if your skills set can rebirth itself into a niche market.

Sometimes markets surge for no apparent reason; masses of people suddenly want something, and the resulting demand can't be immediately met. For example, during the swine flu epidemic there was a huge demand for facial masks in several countries. A trend is also created by larger social movement. As the Golden Boomer market moves towards retirement, there is increased demand for positive ageing. Look at existing wellness businesses and determine if there's a need for more of those products or services.

Once you find a viable niche, learn as much as you can from it. Read and watch the news, keep up with current events and new fads. Watch the industry news. Subscribe to trend sites.

When you spot a possible niche, research the current offerings and size of the market to see if a new business in this niche would be viable. Is the niche underserved? A wellness coaching practice will grow faster in an underserved arena than in a highly developed one that has many vendors trying to meet the given need.

Is there an intense, perceived need for the niche in the minds of your prospects? Are they truly concerned about the issue which you can help them solve with your wellness coaching? The more intense their pain or attractive the benefit, the more quickly the niche will respond to your efforts.

DOES YOUR SKILLS SET GO WITH THE TRENDS?

Based on your research, consider if your skills set goes with the possible niche trends. If so, move ahead. If not, what trends have emerged as part of your research, and where do you think you could fit in with further training?

> ### Inside tip
>
> Have a passion for your niche! Are these the kinds of clients you would enjoy working with? Would you find the work satisfying? Note: often you cannot answer this question in the abstract. Sometimes you must first interact with people in the niche, for example by offering a workshop before you begin to feel the passion stirring. It is not always sufficient to be highly compensated. The niche must be meaningful for you.

Invent a new product or service

Was there a huge demand for retirement coaching 30 years ago? No. The key to coming up with business ideas for a new product or service is to identify a market need that's not being met. Breaking down gay-pride boundaries led to an explosion of new services, such as civil partnership coaching. Look around and ask how can you improve this situation. Focus on a particular target market and brainstorm business ideas for services which the group would be interested in. Ries and Ries (1998) put forward the argument for picking a niche where you are first. You could do this by taking a successful coaching niche and niching it down even more. For example, if you have experience of working with sixth formers, you can narrow the niche and be the first to coach hearing-impaired sixth formers to prepare for university.

What about getting some ideas for wellness-related niche products? Visit www.amazon.com/gp/new-releases to get some inspiration, or take a look at www.google.com/trends.

Add value to an existing product

The difference between chamomile growing in a pot and a tincture of chamomile is a good example of putting a product through an additional process to increase its value. You might also add services, or combine the product with other products. For instance, a herbalist offering consultations and medicinal herbal products also offers coaching for those who want to create herbal gardens. What business ideas can you develop along these lines? Focus on what products you might buy and what you might do to them or with them to create a profitable business.

Improve an existing product or service

There are very few wellness products or services that can't be improved. Start generating business ideas by looking at the products and services you use and identifying ways as to how they could be better.

> ## Inside tip
>
> Creating a niche means digging deeper into what sets your wellness coaching product or service apart from the competition. Look at your location, hours of operation, years of experience, price point, availability, response time to client inquiries or processing orders, the quality of your product or delivery of your service, personalized attention, etc.
>
> Finding your niche is often a matter of putting a new spin on what you already do. Ask yourself: How can I differentiate my business from others? How can I create the perception that my market cannot survive without me. What do I have to offer? What new service or products can I create? For example, the qualification courses I offer are delivered on a one-to-one basis, when the student wants and will also include bespoke options. I offer bespoke CPD options which students can take at any time and covers any special content. Most qualification and CPD courses are offered in a group setting with a start and finish date and set content.
>
> Decide who you want your clients to be. Examine the needs of your clients. Match what you're selling to what the client wants to buy. Make sure your niche is special, unlike anything else out there.

Identifying precedents

Are there already successful businesses in your identified niche? If there are, this may suggest that people are already paying money to have a specific need addressed. This in turn indicates that the market may be more responsive to marketing than if the niche has never been explored. Established or new niches could work. But some of the risk is reduced if you know there are others that are successfully targeting the niche.

Will the client pay for the niche?

Can your prospective clients pay for your services? Wellness coaching may be seen as essential if addressing a condition, but in general it is a discretionary spend, meaning that it isn't as essential as paying the mortgage. Can your target buyers afford your fees? Will they pay? A niche comprised of single parents, for example, might not have much income to spare. A professional niche may easily be able to pay while taking the coaching as a business expense.

Coherent niche

It's useful if members of your proposed niche feel they belong to a coherent group. It's advantageous if as you specialize in the niche, buyers can say, 'This wellness coach lives in my world. They clearly understand my issues.'

Short- or long-term wellness coaching

Is the niche's need for your services short term or enduring? If your niche is general wellness coaching for oil riggers, the window of need of an individual might be short term. Other niches may be more long term, for example wellness coaching for a chronic condition. Remember, it's easier to serve existing clients than to have to continually acquire new ones.

Partnership niche

You might consider developing a new niche with a business partner while sharing costs, creating ideas and supporting each other. You could partner with someone who had profound experience of a niche, 'covering' you while you get up to speed. You could partner with an already successful coach, helping them enlarge the reach of their niche.

Inside tip

Questions to ask yourself when considering a wellness niche:

- Is your coaching niche viable for this economy?
- Is the group accessible?
- Do you know exactly where to find them?
- Do you know exactly what's standing in the way of their success?
- Do they have the disposable income to invest in your solutions?

Niche market ideas

Children/young people

You could offer wellness coaching, workshops and products to schools, clubs and young people around issues of sexual health, healthy eating, self esteem, drugs awareness, bullying, bereavement, depression, substance abuse, stress, phobias, eating disorders, communication skills, conflict management, relationships, life skills, negative emotions, weight management, smoking and body image.

Consider creating a range of one-off coaching workshops or a series of micro-coaching workshops to schools and clubs which can be put together in a specific programme, for example 'Relationship Skills for Young People'.

Don't forget to target those who work with children and young people. You could offer one-to-one and group coaching to teachers, student teachers, family centre workers, classroom assistants and youth workers, coaching them in specific wellness-related skills which would enhance their work.

Then you have the parents. You could offer one-to-one and group coaching in parenting skills or skills to cope with specific wellness issues. There is also a coaching market for family breakdown, separation and divorce.

Wellness-related products could be aimed at those who work with children and young people for them to use in their work.

Women

Women are a massive market for wellness coaching. You could separate the market segments by:

- age; e.g. young women, midlife women, women in retirement
- profession
- hormone status; e.g. PMS, pregnancy, perimenopausal, menopausal
- health issue; e.g. breast cancer, PCOS, etc.
- sexuality; e.g. heterosexual, bisexual, lesbian, transgender
- wellness-related interest; e.g. fitness, nutrition, sexuality, weight
- status; e.g. professional, stay-at-home mum, divorced, single, widowed, separated.

From these segments, you have coaching niches such as weight management for the busy professional, fitness for women in retirement, women recovering from breast cancer, midlife weight management, dating skills for the 30-something woman, young women with PCOS, or first-time pregnancy.

You can offer one-to-one and coaching circles for specific markets. Don't forget your niche market product range.

Men

Men tend to be more cautious about dealing with wellness issues. It is often under duress from someone else or as a last resort that a man will come to wellness coaching. The trick is to present the concept in short, sharp sound bites loaded with practical outcomes. You could separate the market segments by:

- age; e.g. young men, midlife men, men in retirement
- profession
- status; e.g. professional, divorced, single, widowed, separated
- health issue; e.g. prostate cancer, cardiovascular health, erectile dysfunction, etc.
- sexuality; e.g. heterosexual, bisexual, gay, transgender
- wellness-related interest; e.g. fitness, nutrition, sexuality, weight.

From these segments, you could develop wellness coaching niches in, for example, fitness for men over 50, andropause (the male equivalent to menopause), midlife career transition, etc.

Image

Personal appearance says a great deal about a person and makes an indelible first impression, before a word is spoken. As an image coach, you can coach clients in not only improving their appearance but also how they feel about themselves. Image coaching usually involves colour, style and make-up. For an integrated package, you might add building self-esteem and communication skills.

Possible niches could include image coaching for interviews, after mastectomy, young people, retirement, the self-employed, public speakers, the larger man/woman, the pregnant woman, the petite woman, weight management, the tall man/woman, the disabled or for dating.

Image coaching is a nice one to do in groups, especially with women or young people. However, one-to-one is good for many and can incorporate the more personal side of image building.

There is plenty of scope here for products such as colour-related make-up and accessories, DVDs on how to look good for different shapes and sizes, how to present yourself in front of a group, make-up application, hair care and body language.

Specific/chronic conditions

You could work in a niche area by coaching people one-to-one who have chronic conditions such as MS, ulcerative colitis, Crohn's disease, fibromyalgia, arthritis, diabetes, hypertension, cardiac disease, lupus, kidney disease, phobias, pain or fatigue.

You could add on support groups for the condition, as well as a support coaching service for carers and family. Another idea is to offer a strategic alliance to a support group or organization which specializes in your particular condition.

You could also offer related products such as visualization CDs, nutritional downloads or lifestyle products.

You could offer consultations to businesses and management that want to develop a more inclusive environment and allows for greater retention and motivation of their employees who live with chronic illness.

Employee/corporate wellness

This is a crowded marketplace, one which fluctuates with the economic climate. You could offer one-to-one wellness coaching with different slants which may be paid for by the individual or the organization. You might offer a one-stop shop to include:

- employee-assistance programmes
- onsite employee health screening
- postural assessments
- neck, back and shoulder exercise classes
- employee wellness incentive programmes
- 'lunch 'n' learn' seminars
- health fairs providing health screening and assessments, nutrition tasting table (healthy foods), ergonomics, massage/reflexology
- health clinics offering nutritional consultation, personal trainer, weight management, smoking cessation.

For a corporate product, you could publish an employee wellness newsletter. You might strike up a strategic business partnership with local gyms and offer staff discounts in the newsletter.

Sports

Wellness coaching niches could include sports conditioning and disability sports. Some other ideas:

- Provide a wellness mentoring service to sport leaders and coaches.
- For disability coaching, offer training in adapted sports and disability-aware coaches, volunteers and teachers across all impairment groups.

- You could focus on providing sports nutrition coaching.

- For sports coaching with children, offer coaching on a one-to-one basis through to mainstream schools, special schools, clubs, charities and organizations.

The web-based wellness centre

Offer a subscription online, where your members can interact with a wellness coach every day. Your wellness site will encourage members to succeed in achieving their wellness goals. Create a high-quality wellness resource by offering them their own online wellness coach that makes it easy to set goals and track progress, demonstrates proper exercise techniques and motivates and engages members wherever they are.

Create your online service so that you can tailor a programme to virtually any topic your client may request, from smoking cessation or stress reduction to full-scale wellness coaching. You are offering members unlimited access to their own wellness coach for a subscription. Through this service, users not only learn what they need to do, but more important they learn how to sustain their new, healthy lifestyles. You, as their wellness coach, provide positive reinforcement, advice, additional information and support at every step.

Mental health coaching

If you have a psychotherapeutic or counselling background, you might consider wellness coaching niches such as lifestyle, independent living, generalized anxiety disorders, agoraphobia, social anxiety or phobias.

Smoking cessation

Coaches who specialize in this category tend to have a hypnotherapy background. Consider your bolt-on products, such as CDs.

Community health

There are many charities, groups and organizations which have funding and work out in the community delivering wellness initiatives. You could sell your wellness coaching services to these bodies and work on a variety of community projects.

> ## Inside tip
>
> I have spent many years as a community tutor working in locations of social deprivation delivering courses and programmes on aspects of wellness. My contract has been with universities who have been awarded funding for delivery. My client base out in the community has been unemployment centres, community centres and social service family centres.

Weight management

To be successful in this niche, you need a nutritional background. A fitness background would also add to your portfolio. NLP, cognitive behavioural experience and hypnotherapy are good therapies to bolt-on. You could offer support groups or coaching circles, as well as weekly classes.

Consider niching such as post-natal weight management, men, eating disorders and young people. You could offer an online weight management club. For the corporate market, you could do breakfast, lunch or after-work weight management coaching sessions. Don't forget the fitness sessions!

Other ideas include fitness classes and fitness DVDs. You could write a recipe book or post downloadable sheets on your site. Thinking of your website: you could have a subscription part for 'Premier Club Members' to whom, for a monthly fee, you offer tele-coaching or e-coaching, plus access to downloadables.

Inside tip

These are the wellness markets I believe are set to grow and could lend themselves superbly to wellness coaching:

- fitness-based: micro group fitness (training in small groups of two to five), aero jumping (professional boxer Michael Olajide Jr. came up with the idea of a plan which works in the tradition of rope jumping to workout songs that boost your mood and energy), piloxing (combines features of Pilates with boxing), kangoo jumps (pogo jogging shoes combined with a well-defined exercise plan), strength training, Pilates (back problems, post surgery rehabilitation, post pregnancy firming and strengthening, postural correction, etc.), midlife exercise, yoga

- mature learner study coach (huge numbers of people are going back to school – ducking the bad economy, retraining for new jobs)

- integration of spa treatments with wellness specialisms, e.g. nutritionists and targeted activities to create an overall health enhancing experience while using indigenous treatments using local ingredients

- healthy ageing/positive ageing/active ageing/mindful ageing (focus on disease prevention and health enhancement)

- male health (restorative programmes that help with stress reduction and rebalancing)

- non-surgical/non-chemical (beauty) treatments

- wellness through nature (fitness, activities, meditation as part of stress reduction, and treatments, e.g. hiking in the mountains, yoga in the gardens, walks in nature, natural locations for treatments, fitness programmes that encompass outdoor activities).

Spirituality

Regardless of the array of religions and world views, the one mainstay of religion is the unification of body and spirit, the uniting of the human spirit with the belief in a higher power. As mentors in a particular theological perspective, spiritual coaches aid clients through individual religious processes.

> ## Inside tip
>
> Some more wellness markets which are set to grow and could lend themselves to wellness coaching:
>
> - generation Y (teenagers and young adults)
> - specific industry segment (identifying high-stress occupations)
> - intimate relationships
> - Golden Boomers (coaching through later-life transition)
> - weight management
> - condition-led, e.g. heart care
> - nutrition-based, e.g. relaxing and energizing foods, immunity-enhancing foods, healthy sustainable eating (grow your own)
> - holiday-based, e.g. tailor-made gastronomic courses combined with holidays, eco cruises or special interest cruises with well-being as a focus
> - blending wellness with sustainability and green living.

Beauty

You may wonder what beauty is doing under wellness coaching niches. Consider that health and beauty can be linked, giving rise to wellness coaching niches such as healthy skin, detoxing, weight management, managing birth marks and positive ageing.

A nutritional background is helpful. Other therapies which are useful include relaxation, meditation and fitness.

Fitness

The fitness market is booming. Blending personal training with nutritional coaching is a winner. Don't leave out the mindbody link and bolt-on sport NLP. Add in drop-in classes or one-to-one coaching in Pilates or yoga, and away you go.

You might want to specialize in a particular kind of sport, offering sports massage and injury rehabilitation. Do athletic coaching such as strength and conditioning for your sport, postural and biochemical coaching, positive mental performance coaching (using NLP and hypnotherapy).

You could offer specialized coaching programmes such as fitness for pre- and post-natal women. You could offer fitness boot camps on 'Get Fit for Summer' or the 'New Year Fat Burn'. If you work for a gym, run a coaching workshop on specialist equipment or exercise trend. Specialize in coaching people for charity fitness events. Consider the corporate fitness market for physical fitness and team building.

Offer online coaching and training plans.

Inside tip

Students often ask me how I find my wellness coaching niches. There are three key influences to this answer:

1. I believe that who we are gives rise to what we do, and many of my core values and beliefs are represented in the work I choose.

2. My wellness career has evolved partially as a result of my own psychological and physical journeys.

3. I have a belief that people with certain issues gravitate to certain therapist, not only because the therapist has marketed to a particular sector but in an energetic sense.

Retreats and holidays

Don't forget the boom market of fitness and wellness holidays. You can either organize and run one completely yourself or approach hotels and travel companies and strike up a strategic business partnership.

Travel with wellness coach

You'll need to be foot-lose and fancy-free for this niche idea. This is a bespoke service where you accompany an individual or group in order for them to either initiate a healthier lifestyle or stay fit and healthy during a business/private trip. You could include exercise and fitness, yoga and meditation, nutritional guidance plus complementary therapies. Meal design and menu choice plus wellness coaching could all be incorporated into the travel arrangements.

Stress management

Stress-management coaching can be applied to the domestic and corporate market. You could offer one-to-one and group wellness coaching on: work/life balance; work-related stress management relaxation sessions; neck, back and shoulder exercise classes; anger management; conflict resolution; assertiveness coaching; heart health; anxiety management; stress resilience; performance management; and lifestyle awareness.

Research conditions that are stress-related or exacerbated by stress and coach stress-management techniques as part of integrated healthcare.

Ergonomics

Ergonomics is the science of designing user interaction with equipment and workplaces to fit the user and is used to fulfil the two goals of health and productivity. Ergonomics is relevant in the design of such things as safe furniture and easy-to-use machine interfaces in both domestic and work settings.

Coaching activities might include techniques to minimize physical stresses and associated discomfort, and exercises that prevent and minimize discomfort and ergonomic problems.

Products might include reports with recommendations and suggestions for improvement, relevant ergonomics education, and information on how to adjust and work with existing equipment and the environment.

Addiction recovery

Recovery coaching specializes in working with people in recovery from addiction, for example smoking cessation, weight loss, over-eating, Internet, workaholics, gambling, drugs, relationships, alcoholism, problem drinking and sex addiction. The wellness coach would normally have a psychotherapeutic or counselling background.

Time management

A time management coach provides a third-party approach to organizing and prioritizing work and personal objectives by developing useful strategies to effectively use time. I suggest using remote coaching to deliver this one!

Meditation

Combine meditation with relaxation coaching and you have a potentially wide market – for example, pregnancy and birthing, phobia management and exam stress.

Pregnancy/mums

This niche has four potential parts: fertility and pre-conception care, pregnancy, birth preparation and post-natal recovery. For each stage you might offer various therapies, including nutrition. Fertility coaching could include hypnotherapy as a bolt-on. Pregnancy coaching is – if you'll excuse the pun – a growth area. In France, I am reliably informed, the health services have a culture of getting mums who have birthed back to full fitness – and this trend is beginning to arrive in the UK.

You might want to add on HypnoBirthing, Active Birth and baby massage.

Parenting

Adjusting to a parent's lifestyle can be a difficult transition for many people. You could offer coaching to the parents on parenting skills or family wellness. Your market could come from mums, dads, single parents, divorced parents, step-parents, foster parents, expectant parents, first-time parents, teen parents, parents of teens, parents of gifted children, parents of children with special needs, custodial grandparents, parents of blended families, parents with an empty nest, working parents or stay-at-home parents.

The niches they could be interested include health, child behaviour issues, ADD/ADHD, quality of life balance and communication or interpersonal skills.

Positive ageing

With society being somewhat anti-ageing, there is vast potential for working with Golden Boomers and those who have issues with growing older. Some niche ideas: weight loss, dating, career change, balancing care of family (children and parents) and career, finding deeper meaning in life and sexual health.

You can break down these niches further to men or women, particular age brackets, professionals, retirement, menopause, and more.

Relationships/sexuality/gender

This area of wellness coaching offers a range of opportunities, such as sex coaching, coaching for gays and lesbians and relationship coaching.

Niche areas could be dating skills, confidence with women or men, self-confidence and body image issues, better communication in intimate relations, commitment resistance, how to avoid repeating destructive relationship patterns, managing conflict or post-natal sexual recovery for women.

Nutrition

Nutrition is one of few therapies that lends itself very clearly to coaching. Needless to say, you need to be a qualified nutritionist or dietician for this area. You may want to specialize in eating disorders in young people, specific conditions, eating disorders in men, raw food or weight management. These sessions can be delivered through one-to-one and group coaching, on- and offline. You could also offer nutrition-related courses and retreats. Products could abound here, from kitchenware through to specialist or organic foods, as well as DVDs showing the viewer how to prepare a dish. You could have a subscription part of your site where members get access to recipes and other high-value information.

Ethnic communities

People who come from countries with a very different cultures and environments than the UK may experience difficulties acclimatizing and can present with issues around physiological and psychological health which need sensitive handling.

Golden Boomers

Golden Boomers are born between the mid 1940s and the mid 1960s; the first wave is now coming up to retirement age. In the UK, Golden Boomers hold approximately 80 per cent of the wealth; there are 76 million Golden Boomers in the US.

This sector is interested in simplifying their lifestyle, elder-care issues, social and environmental issues, managing time, financial management, later life relationships, maintaining healthy habits, getting enough exercise, smoking cessation, healthy eating, work and career development and time for self. Any of these areas could provide a wellness coaching niche.

Creating a diverse business model

As you already have an existing therapeutic practice, you are looking for developmental opportunities to expand your business to including wellness coaching. The 21st-century healthcare professional creates a business model which has multiple streams of income.

Coaching

This can be done one-to-one or through groups. Both can be done face-to-face and through remote coaching.

Inside tip

As both a therapist and a coach, I have found one of the most useful marketing approaches is to be condition-led rather than technique-led. People tend to respond to the problem rather than the methodology.

Health promotion

Health promotion differs from education inasmuch as health promotion is more a 'talking at' rather than the interactive approach that education and training offer. Normally this is done in groups, but it could lead to private work. You could aim your health promotion work at the domestic or corporate market.

Screening

As part of your wellness services, you may want to offer tests or screening. Screening might already be part of your therapeutic work. Or you could also offer it as part of, for example, a 'Corporate Wellness Day'.

Inside tip

When I was 28 and began my wellness practice (over 20 years ago), I started to do astrological readings and taught self-development courses like assertiveness training, etc., for my local AE college. I added on a private coaching practice and took on one-to-one clients who came from the AE courses.

I moved on to running wellness-related courses across all sectors, such as prisons, FE, HE, corporate, community education and private clients.

Then I started to add the therapies. First, reflexology. I realized many problems were caused by poor diet. I added nutrition. Lots of stress-related issues presented. I added stress-management therapy. For me, a spiritual perspective was needed to underlie the practical healing process. In went Reiki. Throughout the journey, I bolted on flower essences, training in cognitive behavioural interventions, and more besides. I've always tried not to add similar therapies. Rather I've created a weave of eclectic approaches. In fact, most of my clients come to me because of the eclectic approach.

I provide therapy and coaching through one-to-one and group work. If someone doesn't want to see me personally, we talk on the phone or email. If they don't want any personal contact, I sell them a product. Always have an angle you can offer.

Consultancy

A consultant (from the Latin *consultare*, meaning 'to discuss') is a professional who provides expert advice in a particular area of expertise. In your case, the expertise is wellness or a specific condition or healthcare method. A consultant is a knowledge worker. This could be a good route if you are marketing to the corporate or business-to-business sector. Follow these steps to decide whether consultancy is right for you:

1. Audit your work history and list all the key projects you've undertaken over the years: your knowledge, skills and experience. What did you do, and what was the outcome? Summarize this into a set of areas where you can provide useful and powerful insights to others. Ask yourself, 'What have I learned in my career that I can sell to others?' This becomes your product.

2. Ask yourself whether your list of knowledge areas is valued by the marketplace. Ideally you want the skills you're offering to match a growing area of demand. Consider the health-related sectors in which you want to develop consultancy work. What are the trends here? What are people talking about in relation to wellness and health consultancy? Where's demand rising and falling? Are the type and style of offerings changing? Who are the movers and shakers in the area? Research economic growth potential. Look to the national press, TV, adverts, Internet, films, music, magazines, even food fashions – all of these can help inform you of social trends. And don't forget all the readily accessible research data from public, educational and commercial sources. Regularly review related journals and press, health-related publishers' new lists, and conference and seminar promotional materials to discover popular topics.

3. Once you've analyzed your marketplace, overlay the skills and experience you plan to offer against these trends, and assess whether there will be sufficient demand for your expertise in the consultancy area that you can target.

4. One of the most important aspects of establishing and marketing yourself as a consultant is developing a product set. Clients like to buy something specific. You want to be seen as specialist, expert and knowledgeable. So package your expertise into products that clients understand and recognize. A well-packaged product concept for which you've identified a market need is far easier to consume than some generalized expertise. You may be able to offer the generalized expertise later, off the back of a successful product sale.

Training

You may want to offer workshops and courses around various aspects of wellness. You could offer bespoke wellness training to the corporate market, or deliver public courses to the business sector which are open to everyone. You might want to focus on the domestic market and run courses for specific target groups such as family wellness. From training might come private work.

Complementary therapies

It is assumed, as you are reading this book, that you are already a therapist of some kind. It is always good to have a range of integrated complementary therapies to offer clients alongside wellness coaching.

Inside tip

As a teacher of accredited health and wellness-related courses, I meet many people: some who are just starting out on their career and others who have a great deal of experience behind them.

For those just starting out: while it is important to add new knowledge and skills through further training, don't avoid the real world by taking yet another course. It is crucial that you start to deliver your service as soon as possible. You need experience and confidence building more than another certificate!

For those experienced therapists, while it is important to continue CPD, don't blind your clients with an array of confusing therapies. Maybe it's your business skills that need honing rather than your therapeutic skills!

Retreats and holidays

Wellness tourism is a booming area with an average buyer aged 44. People want to escape from everyday life and tend to be cash-rich and time-poor. They have a desire to simplify and slow down life or to search for like-minded people. Other reasons for the growth in this industry is a need to improve the self with balance and integration. Other travellers are on a spiritual quest, seek recuperation, or wish to travel to inspirational landscapes.

There is a rise in condition-led workshops and treatments. Girlie weekend packages and mother/daughter packages are popular. Customized products and services and 'signature' treatments are called for (if you offer spa or complementary health treatments, consider creating your signature package). We've seen an increase in corporate wellness. Breaks that provide local and indigenous products go down well. Other interesting growth markets are in wellness treatments for animals and creative/art therapy. Spa and wellness cruises are popular, especially spas offering education and lifestyle programmes such as preventative healthcare, fitness regimes, gastro, detox or healthy eating. There is a rise in teenage and male spa users.

Wellness tourism areas include:

- Spiritual tourism, e.g. pilgrimage, meditation retreat.
- Occupational wellness tourism, e.g. life coaching, stress management.
- Traditional spa, where you sit in mineral waters, have a massage or sauna or enjoy the steam room. These tend to appeal to older people with specific conditions.
- Hotel and day spa: Think beauty treatment, relaxing massage, aromatherapy and jaccuzi. Motivations are cosmetic, relaxing and pampering and tend to draw from high-income women or business tourists.
- Purpose-built recreational spa: These complexes include swimming pools, thermal waters, themed saunas/steam rooms, jaccuzis and fitness activities. They appeal for physical conditions and relaxation.
- Seaside resorts/thalassotherapy: These resorts cover hydrotherapy, salt inhalations, salt scrubs, seaweed wraps and tanning for physical, curative and cosmetic reasons. They usually appeal to high-income, older buyers.
- Holistic retreats: Think yoga, massage, creative, spiritual and psychological workshops. The motivation is usually physical, mental, psychological, social, creative and spiritual wellness. The market is likely to be female Golden Boomers aged 35–55.
- Yoga and meditation centres: These centres cover yoga, meditation, chanting and fasting activities for physical, mental and spiritual reasons. They appeal to 40-something Golden Boomers, hippies and professional women.
- Pilgrimage centres: These breaks appeal to mainly the under-30-somethings and are for visiting spiritual landscapes, religious buildings and walking pilgrimage routes. They are not necessarily religious-based.
- Medical centres: These tend to be for operations, cosmetic surgery, dentistry or special treatments and appeal to 30-something Western Europeans and Americans for whom treatment is cheaper abroad.

You might want to form a strategic business partnership with a retreat centre or hotel with spa facilities and offer a specific type of break – or you might want to run the whole kit and caboodle.

Information products

These are wellness-related products which you can sell through your website or clinic, or give away free. Information products can be repackaged in different ways; for example, have your CDs transcribed and turned into articles, e-books or special reports. Turn your e-books into membership programmes using an autoresponder service.

BOOKLETS

Booklets on specific conditions or aspects of wellness coaching are useful as a client memory aid. If you work with back problems, you could compile a booklet of useful exercises. You could team the booklet up with a DVD showing the exercises in action. You could use the booklet as a freebie but sell the DVD and booklet together.

ARTICLES

Articles build your expertness in the eyes of the reader. For example, you could put a couple of articles up on your site related to packing nutritious lunchboxes for kids. You would place a couple of articles on sites which attract parents, like 'Lowering Your Child's Fat Intake in 3 Easy Steps' (and always remember to have that link back to your site). There is unlikely to be money in articles, unless you're a professional writer, but they will drive visitors to your site who might become buyers.

E-ZINES

An e-zine is a really easy way to keep visitors to your site informed of new happenings, such as discounted therapies, new workshops or free health-related resources. By offering a free e-zine (maybe with the hook of a free information product), you can capture their emails and entice them back to your website through your regular e-zine.

NEWSLETTERS

A newsletter is similar to an e-zine but is more in-depth. While an e-zine might inform, a newsletter takes the reader deeper into a particular subject. For example, if you teach an offline course, 'Homeopathy for Children' (which you could turn into an information product via an online course), you might want to include an article in your newsletter called 'How to Use Homeopathy for Sleep Problems with Children'. You could also use this as an article on your site and on related sites, such as those that offer advice for children.

TUTORIALS

What about offering short online courses? You might choose to charge and support the learner or you could offer it as a free resource without any tutor support. If you are a counsellor, for example, you might want to offer a short tutorial called 'How to Overcome Shyness in Social Situations'.

COURSES

A course is similar to tutorials, but longer. You could offer this online (email) or distance (post) or face-to-face. You would need to offer student support.

DVD

You can make a short how-to video or DVD on a specific subject and sell it as online and offline to your clients. For instance 'DIY Foot Massage' or 'Acupressure for Headaches and Migraine'.

CD

For example, if you specialize in stress-management techniques, why not create a short relaxation techniques audio CD and sell it online, or create MP3 or WAV files to download? Make up a booklet and you could sell the package to clients in your clinic.

TRAINING MANUALS

Do you have any learning material you could turn into training products to sell to trainers? Could you sell short self-study courses online with the same material?

SOFTWARE

If you are computer wiz-kid and have health-related experience, you could create client management software for healthcare professionals or create a piece of software to guide people through, for example, 'Managing Your Own Weight Loss Programme'.

Inside tip

To build a thriving 21st-century wellness practice, offer information products. You're in business to make money, but there are two types of information products which I would suggest you offer *free* through your website:

E-books
If you have extensive knowledge on an aspect of healthcare or wellness, create an e-book.

Reports
Creating a short, downloadable report. Research will raise your profile as an expert in health and wellness.

These information products will increase visitors to your site, establish your credibility and build your reputation. If you offer a new e-book or report, say every three months, your freebie lookers may turn into cash buyers. In order for someone to download your information product, ask for their email address. Then you can build your database for your wellness e-zine.

Your five-step plan to finding your wellness coaching niche

1. Identify a niche possibility, paying attention to the groups that naturally turn to you for help as well as those groups to which you've had some work or personal experience and exposure. Consider pairing a speciality with a business market. For example:

    a. working with executive women to manage their stress levels

    b. helping solo entrepreneurs to build their business around their lifestyle choices, rather than the other way around.

2. Consider the following:

    a. your personal investment:

        i. How does the niche encourage your authenticity?

        ii. How does the niche reflect your values?

        iii. How does the niche inspire your interest level?

    b. your current skills and knowledge:

        i. What is your professional track-record with regard to the niche?

      ii.   What is your qualification background with regard to the niche?

   c. the identified client base:

      i.   How can you get to the identified client base?

      ii.   How willing is the identified client base to pay for the niche coaching?

      iii. Who is the competition?

      iv. What is the growth potential of the niche?

3. If you decide to proceed with your niche idea, move into research. Interview several prospects to better identify:

   a. what their greatest needs are

   b. how to best communicate to the niche

   c. what your competition looks like

   d. how to quickly position yourself as an expert to the niche

   e. how to best package your coaching as a solution to the niche's greatest unmet, tangible needs that they are prepared to pay money to resolve.

By 'package', I mean arrange your coaching in tangible parcels, for example six months of one-to-one coaching with specific content (things they will learn), workshops, tele-classes, webinars, etc.

4. Test market your solution. Create a programme, e.g. one-to-one, tele-classes, workshops, etc. to try out your coaching solution, gain testimonials, and learn more about your niche. Sometimes you may have to almost give away your first programme, but it will be worth it. You will learn so much more about what of your material works and what doesn't, and what other needs the niche may have. And the testimonials from the participants in your pilot programme will be invaluable in future selling.

5. Roll out your finished product while seeking every opportunity to speak, write, present and share your knowledge with your target audience to increase your exposure and solidify your position as an expert solution provider to this niche. The greater the expert profile you have with the group, the more responsive they will be to your invitation to participate in your programme.

CPD task sheet

This is your Continuing Professional Development (CPD) task sheet which summarizes key module points and offers you the opportunity to engage with tasks to deepen your learning.

Module summary

- It is important to create a niche in order to focus on an accessible and productive market and to build your expertise and kudos in the opinion of that market.

Your task

Follow the five-step plan to identify two niche markets for your wellness coaching.

Applying Wellness Coaching

By the end of the module, you will have explored:

- Five ways to deliver wellness coaching
- Information products

Five ways to deliver wellness coaching

You've chosen your wellness niches. What are the various ways you can deliver?

Method 1: Individual face-to-face coaching

Individual face-to-face wellness coaching sessions usually last for one to two hours and are paced out over weeks or months. You might meet with your client weekly, fortnightly or monthly. It can occur on your premises, within a group clinic environment, on the client's premises or in neutral territory such as a rented office or hotel lounge. Many coaches offer packages which are pre-paid for in advance. Or you could offer coaching on an ad hoc basis.

This way of coaching is up front and personal, and makes for a more intense coaching experience. The interaction includes the subtlety of body language as well as content. If you are on your own premises, you can deliver a treatment, if appropriate. On the downside, clients might feel put on the spot with face-to-face coaching – there's nowhere to run. Also, there is the risk your client might not turn up. From your perspective, even if you're having a bad hair day, you still need to put on your glad-rags and smile.

> ## Inside tip
>
> I find that with face-to-face coaching I can get a more complete picture of the client. There is more scope for interpreting the nuances of body language and building rapport.
>
> In my coaching room I have a wealth of interactive resources for clients to use, and there is plenty of opportunity to coach them through creative hands-on tasks. Also activities such as role-play can only really happen in a face-to-face situation.

Method 2: Laser coaching

Many people put off wellness coaching because they're afraid of the time commitment. They fear weekly one-hour appointments stretching on indefinitely, and because of this, miss out on the benefits of a wellness coach. Laser coaching removes the fear of long-term commitment. With laser coaching, clients hone down their concerns to one bite-sized piece that can be addressed in a one- or two-hour session. Client and coach work intensively in that time and emerge with an action plan. No further sessions are necessary. Additional laser coaching on different topics can always be added without ongoing commitment. Laser coaching works best in the following situations:

- The client has one or two defined concerns but is otherwise confident about their wellness.

- A client wants to check out a coach before making a long-term commitment. Starting with one or two laser-coaching sessions is a good way to make sure you can work together.

- The problem involves the immediacy of a wellness issue. Laser coaching can quickly help develop skills for dealing with the here-and-now.

- The problem is part of a larger issue that can be broken into smaller related pieces. For example, a client who gets stressed over public speaking may choose to deal with that anxiety over a series of laser-coaching sessions spread out at his convenience, as budget permits. By breaking a big topic into smaller pieces, it's possible to make progress without a long-term coaching commitment.

The client should come prepared with a clearly defined wellness-related issue and objective. Laser coaching makes sense as a time-efficient and cost-effective way to get results.

> ## Inside tip
>
> I've done a lot of laser coaching. It is a popular option and, providing you keep the session on track, a lot can be accomplished. A downside can be if you get clients who drone on. Then you may find yourself constantly pulling them to the focus of the session. Some people can come in with high expectations of the session; e.g. they want their IBS and marriage sorted in one hit.

Method 3: Group coaching

This method of delivery involves facilitating and coaching several participants at the same time. You might do this via an open workshop (anyone can attend) or through a targeted group, such as social workers on a stress-management coaching programme.

WORKSHOPS

Workshops can vary in length from two hours to two days, or even longer. By definition, it is a practical, hands-on learning experience which is skill based.

Workshops are popular among participants because they are cost effective, social and offer a forum to share ideas. Participants share their skills and learn from each other, and leave the workshop with a set of skills they can build on. They have access to an expert (you!), and motivation usually increases in a group environment. You need to be good at managing group dynamics: for example, the withdrawing participant, the blabbering participant, etc. It can be difficult to give individual attention, and you might find break-times filled with participants wanting your expertise – free!

From your perspective, there is a plethora of pros: the more participants, the higher your fee; it opens the way for one-to-one client work; and your profile is raised.

Here are the necessary steps to get your one-day workshop happening:

1. Identify your market

Is your target market professional (i.e., corporate), work-related or domestic (public)? What wellness needs are you addressing through your workshop? How would you describe your target participant? What would the benefits be to your target participant; e.g. what awareness, knowledge or skills will they acquire, and how will this benefit their work or life? How are these needs currently being addressed? What gap could your workshop fill?

2. Define workshop objectives

An *objective* is an outcome that a participant is expected to achieve by the end of your workshop, e.g. the ability to use simple breathing techniques (skill) to manage anxiety, or understanding (knowledge) how self-esteem affects performance. List six objectives for your workshop based on the needs identified from your target market.

3. Organize the workshop

Consider the timing for the workshop. Weekday or weekend? What time factors should you take into account for your target market? Where will the workshop be held? Consider disabled access and parking. Make sure the room is what you require. If your target market is young people, doctors, people coming to learn meditation or executives, your learning space needs to reflect their expectations. Do you provide the learning resources such as a whiteboard or flipchart, or are these items provided with the room? Don't forget access to power points for computer functions. Are you providing refreshments? Are there kitchen facilities to use? Are there eating places nearby?

4. Market the workshop

Having identified your target market, how are you going to reach them? How far in advance do you need to begin reaching them? What administration procedures do you need in place to enroll participants and to take payment?

5. Design the workshop

Design your workshop to achieve your objectives. Here is a rough outline for an interactive-style workshop:

1. Welcome participants.

2. Explain domestics: fire exits, loos, etc.

3. Everyone introduces self or another; you could blend this with an ice-breaker.

4. Introduce a topic, move into discussion, facilitate small group activity and bring back the whole group for discussion.

5. Move into other topics, depending on time, and allow for a mid-morning break.

6. After lunch, start with an energizer.

7. Introduce a topic, move into discussion, facilitate small group activity, bring back the whole group for discussion.

8. Move into other topics, depending on time, and allow time for a mid-afternoon break.

9. Move into closure and summarizing of day, asking participants to do an evaluation.

10. Bring closure to the workshop.

Include a variety of activities and build in plenty of feedback time. Use handouts or create a participant workbook to use throughout the day.

6. Deliver the workshop

You need to open and close the day, and you need to introduce each topic and set the criteria for activities. In between, you are the facilitator and holder of the learning space for participants to explore and experience. Clarify participants' understanding throughout. Be observant and available and keep the day moving.

7. Evaluate the workshop

At the end of the workshop, the participants need to complete an evaluation sheet. Based on this, you can implement improvements and pat yourself on the back for successes. Don't forget to complete an evaluation process from your perspective.

Inside tip

Many a wellness coaching workshop has passed under my belt, delivered to both the public and private sector. Most people value the support of others who have the same problem. Some, however, look for access to an expert while 'hiding' behind the group identity. Be mindful that the coaching session doesn't turn into a therapy session. However, if you hold the group well, participants go away with a good knowledge set and practical skills they can use. Of course, you don't know what they will do with this newly acquired opportunity. Some will do nothing. Others might do something and get it a bit wrong. Mostly, you won't know. To counter this, you could offer discounted one-to-one follow-up sessions or ongoing group coaching.

Method 4: Tele-coaching

INTRODUCTION TO REMOTE COACHING

Remote coaching is when you are not in the same room as the person you are coaching. At times like this, you would be coaching by telephone, email or webcam.

Remote coaching is becoming the norm and is proving to be effective and efficient. Wellness coaches have the opportunity to do more impromptu coaching and make check-in calls with their clients to build accountability, reinforce a message, handle a challenge or celebrate a success. This 'just in time' coaching can now be delivered when your client needs it most. Remote coaching is cost effective for both you and your client. There are no travel hassles (making international clients possible) and the coaching is accessible anywhere there is a phone or Internet connection. There are no room-hire costs. With tele-coaching and e-coaching, you can deliver in your pyjamas! The downside can be the lack of dynamic in-person human interaction.

Whether you are coaching face-to-face or remotely, the same tools, strategy and coaching framework still work, are applicable and are just as effective, regardless of the environment in which you are coaching.

HOW TO DELIVER TELE-COACHING

Tele-coaching (individual or group) is synchronous, occurring with little or no gap in time between the responses of coach and client.

Some tips for individual tele-coaching:

- Arrange with your clients when they are to call you and how long the sessions will last. Make sure you have client notes, pen and paper before taking the call. Have a clock nearby.

- Start your call with a friendly opening. This could be, 'How is the weather where you are today? Better than here, I hope!' Reply to their answer with a relevant but positive response and then move the call forward: 'That's great, I'm glad you are having a good day. How would you like to use today's session?'

- Agree with the client, before you start, what the session will cover.

- A smiling voice can be heard and is welcoming and relaxing. Your client will subconsciously appreciate it and respond.

- Sit upright, as this helps you to sound enthusiastic and positive (relaxing comfortably tends to make you sound relaxed and comfortable!).

- To create affinity with your callers, speed up or slow down your speaking voice to match theirs.

- Refocus their attention by using their names (and keep doing this if they seem to be losing the plot).

- Take notes as you go.

- Use active listening.

- When you communicate information to your clients, be clear: ask them to repeat back to you how they understand what you've just said. Ask them if they have any questions. When you receive information from your clients, paraphrase every so often to confirm you're following the plot.

- Let other people talk! Make sure your clients have completely finished speaking before responding. Sometimes they haven't finished talking; they are just coming up for air. You listen more effectively when you're not talking, so refrain from interrupting your client.

- Don't pre-empt what your clients are going to say. Chances are you will be wrong and miss some of the content of their conversation.

- Recap key facts. Summarize and reflect back to check you have heard the key facts and content of the client's conversation correctly. This also lets clients know you have understood them. Statements such as 'What I'm hearing is…' and 'Sounds like you are saying…' are great ways to reflect back and summarize.

- You should always talk less than the client.

- Use your words for best results. Keep in mind you can phrase anything positively, negatively or neutrally. Phrasing your words positively will help you get better results more easily.

- Stay focused. Prevent yourself from being distracted and concentrate on what your client is saying.

- Detect emotions. Listen to the emotion in your client's voice. Does it match or endorse the words she is using? Acknowledge any emotions and/or difficulties she's having. Empathy can be shown by using phrases such as 'I can see where you are coming from'.

- Use open-ended questions to get your client to speak more freely. Ask questions to gain more information on points you need to clarify.

- If you are thinking of answers and responses while the client is speaking, you are not listening. If you have difficulty listening, make the necessary adjustments. You might say, 'I'm sorry I missed that last point. Please repeat that for me.'

- Let clients know you are listening by responding with 'um's and 'ah's as they speak.

- Use words that your client uses in her conversation, especially adjectives (words they use to describe something). Example: your client says, 'The results were fab'. In this instance, the word *fab* was chosen because it reflects what the speaker felt. To build rapport, use the same word back at any relevant time: for example, 'I agree with what you said earlier: the results were fab.'

- It is possible to remain professional and still be friendly. This is easily achieved by using good inflection and modulation in your voice, showing an interest in your client's conversation and sharing laughter and lighthearted moments when the opportunity arises during the call.

- Keep a record of what you discussed and any follow-up action that your client (or you) promise to take. Verify this with your client. You might want to confirm your discussions and agreements by a follow-up email.

HOW TO DELIVER TELE-SEMINARS

In addition to individual tele-coaching, you can also offer group tele-coaching through tele-seminars. You could do a one-off tele-seminar or weekly tele-seminars for a set number of weeks. You might be offering wellness-related education or coaching.

Clients call into a bridge line which allows everyone to hear everyone else. As the moderator, you have control to mute the call or not. If the call is muted, only the moderator can speak; if the call isn't muted, anyone can speak.

You need to source a tele-seminar hosting company. Determine what you need and what you can afford. Pick the host company and package that meet your needs and confirm the details in writing. Charges may be by the minute or by participant. Make sure you know what you and the host company are each responsible for. Attend any training the host company offers, and do a practice run before the seminar. Test the equipment and verify that you have access to all required software.

Inside tip

I was approached by a redundancy coach who wanted to do a 50-minute tele-seminar with 12 redundancy/business experts. The punters would come from each expert's mailing list (1000s x 12!) and the tele-seminars would be free to the punter. After the tele-seminars, all 12 'interviews' would be put onto one audio product, which would then be available for each expert to sell to their mailing list.

Decide whether you are going to go for an educational or coaching slant. Decide who should attend. Plan the time, date and length of the tele-seminar. Market the tele-seminar.

Send meeting invitations, confirmations and reminders to participants. Include all key information such as links, log in IDs and passwords, tele-conference phone number and participant code. If you are delivering an education tele-seminar, make an outline for participants so that they can follow you during the call.

Organize an outline for yourself to follow during the tele-seminar of the key points and topics you would like to cover or educate participants about. Be the first to dial in to the tele-seminar.

Greet participants as they join the meeting and introduce yourself. Write down participants' names. As you conduct the tele-seminar, be friendly and engaging. Start the tele-seminar by introducing yourself. Whenever feasible, ask all attendees to introduce themselves to the group. Ask if everyone can hear you speaking. Assist anyone who needs help. Review the tele-seminar agenda and objectives. Set expectations, such as encouraging participation and whether you can accept questions by email or instant messenger. If you are teaching, ask participants to mute their phones to reduce background noise as you conduct the tele-seminar. Constantly demonstrate enthusiasm for your topic. End the tele-seminar on time and thank participants for attending. Provide any follow-up information and resources. Be the last one to hang up.

Inside tip

You can make an information product out of any form of tele-coaching. Offer your clients a recording of the tele-coaching and provide it for their review later. You have your conversation, and end up with an audio file (often an MP3) as a record of your call. Here are a couple of ideas:

- In group tele-seminars, have your seminar recorded as an MP3 to use as a podcast.
- Get a transcription of your call to be used in various ways, e.g. a blog series, an e-book, as the foundation for a guide or manual.

Upload the recorded tele-seminar to your website. Let your clients know that they can also listen to your tele-seminar on your site.

Method 5: Internet coaching (remote coaching)

Internet coaching involves asynchronous (occurs with a gap in time between the responses of coach and client) and synchronous distance interaction among coach and clients using email, chat and video conferencing features.

E-COACHING

E-coaching is delivered over an electronic medium such as email, focuses on the same goals as regular coaching and involves asynchronous distance interaction between coach and client, using text to communicate.

E-coaching is cost effective for you and your client. There are no travel costs, and it can be done from any location. E-coaching gives the client time to consider before answering. There is also opportunity for the wellness coach to refer back to the exact words used, even copying the text to remind clients of what they said earlier. This approach gives more time for a considered dialogue with no time constraints and flexibility. The downside can be that the instinctive responses obtained during tele-coaching or face-to-face are sometimes more genuine.

Inside tip

I have found e-coaching to be best as part of a package with face-to-face or tele-coaching. Some people like the variety of contact methods. Others have a lot to say!

INTERACTIVE TEXT COACHING

Interactive text-based individual and group coaching involves synchronous distance interaction between coach and client using text to communicate.

WEBCAM COACHING

Video-based individual and group Internet coaching involves synchronous distance interaction between coach and clients using what is seen and heard via video to communicate.

Webcam coaching involves a webcam (video camera) whose output is viewed in real time over the Internet. The most popular use is for videotelephony, permitting a computer to act as video conferencing station. This can be used in messenger programmes such as Yahoo!, Windows Live Messenger and Skype messenger services.

Coaches can set up a web-based resource centre to facilitate the Internet coaching process and include interactive scheduling tools, goal-setting tools, learning activities and digital records to record progress.

Internet coaching has many benefits. As it can occur both synchronously and asynchronously, clients can work at more convenient times. It can be more time efficient than regular coaching, as goals can often be achieved much more quickly and in fewer sessions. As a result, Internet coaching is more cost efficient than regular coaching.

Information products

Information products are anything which tells somebody about something. In the Internet context, the term refers to electronically deliverable, knowledge-based products. Some information products are best used as a give-away, while others you could make a good profit from.

You can create wellness-related information products for sale in your clinic or coaching area or via another outlet, online or offline. Benefits of information products can:

- generate passive income (you can earn while you sleep!)
- be reproduced in any quantity
- eliminate shipping cost problems, if delivered electronically
- mitigate the time lapse between purchase and delivery, if delivered electronically.

Complete wellness coaching programmes

People want to learn from someone who has a likable personality and an engaging style. If you start your own wellness coaching programme, you can add your experiences and give the information your own personal flavour through CDs, DVDs and self-help downloadables.

Beginner's guides

Generally speaking, there are usually more beginners than experts, so this is a big market no matter what niche of wellness coaching you choose. You could create a range of beginner how-to guides for your niche.

Reviews

Savvy buyers want to spend their money on the best products and services for the lowest cost. In-depth reviews are high in demand because they fulfil this need. Review and analyze wellness-related products in your niche and sell the information to interested customers.

Expert interviews

Gather the top people in your wellness niche and conduct interviews with each of them. This way, you'll provide a lot of well-rounded content to potential buyers and benefit from the authority and expertise of others. Essentially, you become an expert by association.

Lists of resources

A lot of information is out there on the Internet, and it can get very overwhelming at times. In fact, people are willing to pay for the convenience of having everything they need neatly organized for them – even if everything is freely available online. The time-saving factor is of high value. Compile a list of the best resources for your wellness niche and sell it to people who are looking for the information.

E-books

E-books are easy to create and distribute. As long as you have quality content, PDFs have a higher-perceived value than a blog on a website. Here are the ten steps to writing your own wellness-related e-book:

STEP 1: FORMAT OF THE E-BOOK
PDL, HTML, AZW plain text files, multimedia and Amazon Kindle formats are the most relevant formats for writing an e-book which is then sold to earn an online income. Among these formats, the plain text format is the simplest to use, and multimedia the most complicated one.

STEP 2: IDENTIFY YOUR MARKET
Consider the market to which you want the e-book to appeal.

STEP 3: RESEARCH
Determine the specifics of the content of the e-book.

STEP 4: THE TITLE
Come up with a good title that will catch the attention. The title should give a bird's eye view of what the readers could expect from your e-book.

STEP 5: INTRODUCTION AND CONTENTS PAGE
The introduction is a good way for people to see what you are offering. Every e-book should be preceded by a table of contents telling readers at a glance what they are going to read. This is essential. It should be well organized, neat and be easy for the reader to review.

STEP 6: WRITE THE BOOK
Any e-book 30 or more pages in length should be divided into relevant chapters.

STEP 7: IMAGES
Whatever the content of the e-book, include at least one image for every three pages. Pictures are a visual treat and give an idea about the contents.

STEP 8: EDIT CAREFULLY
Before submitting for publishing, make sure you have edited your e-book carefully.

STEP 9: COLOUR SCHEME
Choosing a colour scheme is the easiest part of writing an e-book. Usually these books are printed on a white background in black print.

STEP 10: CREATING A COVER
One of the main components of an e-book is its cover. It is essential to have a good and well-designed cover page for the e-book, or else people who see it will tend to judge it by its cover and could be put off in the case of its not-so-good appearance.

Reports
One of the most untapped information products is in the creation of small reports (7–15 pages) on specific wellness-related topics, for example:

- 17 Ways to Live a Greener Life
- How to Walk Off 7 Pounds in 7 Days
- 19 Ways to Improve Your Health Free of Charge
- The 15-Minute Guide to a Better Sex Life

There are several further advantages to small report creation: you can sell several reports to one customer, bundle a series of reports into a course, be at the cutting edge when a hot topic emerges or offer a free report to supplement another product or service. The price of a report is likely to be around £5 or so, which is affordable for most people.

Membership sites
A membership site is by far the most flexible information format; it allows you to foster a community on your site and deliver your content in a wide variety of ways, including text, presentation slides, interactive software, video and audio.

You also get the benefit of a continuity model that pays you every month via membership fees.

STEP 1: PICK YOUR WELLNESS-RELATED NICHE MARKET

If you want to build a membership website that will succeed, choose your target market carefully. Avoid going for generic markets like weight loss which already have thousands of membership sites. Instead, focus on a niche market that appeals to a specific category of people. For instance, you can start a membership site for over 50s who want to lose weight.

STEP 2: RESEARCH THE MARKET

Work in social network sites like Facebook and MySpace to connect with users who may be interested in your niche market.

STEP 3: CREATE

It's paramount that you understand what your members want, if you want your site to last. A membership website should be built around people's needs, so it's vital that you conduct thorough research to offer exactly what your members want. The site should include regular updates with high-value content, professional offers, professional testimonials, a blog, regular interaction with members, multimedia, tools and downloads, and automated account set up and reoccurring monthly charges.

Print copies

Print books and publications are still popular today because people want to take them around wherever they go without having to use a computer. You have two choices here. One is to write and self-publish your own books (visit www.inkylittlefingers.co.uk for bespoke options on printing your created books and manuals). All the profit goes to you – and so does all the hard work, including marketing. Option two is to approach book publishers who, if they like your wellness-related book idea, will publish and market your book. (I recommend *Writers' and Artists' Yearbook* for a comprehensive list of publishers in the UK and abroad.) Payment this way comes via royalties, usually a percentage of each book sold.

DVDs and CDs

If you're into multimedia, you might create DVDs and CDs in addition to streaming the files online. People enjoy getting physical products in the mail and are more likely to use them if they have them at hand. This format also gives people the option to use them away from the computer, TV or CD player.

> ## Inside tip
>
> Unless you have excellent recording software, I suggest you use a professional recording studio. When I began recording CDs for wellness, I did it at home. Not so good. So I used a professional recording studio plus engineer who did a superb job. Before recording, you need to write down your script. Then you record. Then the engineer tweaks. Then you re-record various bits you're not keen on. Then you have your master CD to take away. You can burn copies on your computer or get them professionally done in bulk. You can sell the CDs through your website (and others) and in your coaching/clinic area. You can sell them on their own or as part of a bundle.

Email newsletters

You can build up a database of people interested in your services and products from your website. A regular email is then sent to them detailing offers, new services and products, items of interest, etc. Always provide a link back to your site from the newsletter. Also include an opt-out clause so that readers can unsubscribe from the newsletter.

Get your information product happening

- Research demand: Choose a wellness-related topic that you have a passion about, that you know about (or can research) and that people want.

- Identify your target audience: After deciding on a specific topic, segment your potential audience. Do you go for the newbies or the experienced? Young or old? For example, if you want to work with Golden Boomers, there are loads of people under that umbrella with very different needs. Do you want to appeal to men or women? There are premenopausal women, those who want to lose weight, prepare for retirement, look good for potential partners, a change of career, etc. It's not enough to just decide on a topic. You have to identify your target audience and cater to their needs, both in the value you provide and in your marketing.

- Be specific: Once you have a well-researched topic and a target audience, consider a product idea. Be specific, so that your product will be more targeted and relevant with less competition. For example, rather than selling a vague 'Getting through the Perimenopause' guide, create something more targeted like 'The Executive Woman's Guide to Managing Perimenopause'. In doing so, you carve out a specific sub-niche (perimenopause) for your target audience (executive women).

- Decide on what type of product: Are you going to create a written product or an audio or visual product? Will it be online or offline delivery or both?

- Repeat business: Information products are usually not very expensive. Most cost £10 or less, so to build a reliable, long-term business through information products, you have to get your customers coming back for more. Keep this in mind when you create your information product and structure it so that follow-ups and upgrades can be offered.

Inside tip

Don't lose it all because you violated a trademark. Did you know that you can't always show a logo like that of Google in your information product without written consent? You should also run a trademark check on the title of your information product. Visit www.nameprotect.com.

CPD task sheet

This is your Continuing Professional Development (CPD) task sheet which summarizes key module points and offers you the opportunity to engage with tasks to deepen your learning.

Model summary

- Face-to-face coaching, laser coaching, group coaching/workshops, remote coaching (webcam, telephone, email) and information products are all valuable delivery methods for wellness coaching.

Your task

Explore each delivery method to see how it would fit your chosen niche.

Marketing Wellness Coaching

By the end of the module, you will have explored:

- Consumer buying behaviour
- What you are selling
- 62 marketing ideas for wellness coaching
- Creating a wellness coaching marketing plan

Consumer buying behaviour

You've got your product or service. Now you want to sell it. Let's have a look at the process the potential wellness client goes through before making a purchase.

Identifying the problem/need

How do you decide you want to buy a particular product or service? For example, suppose you want extra portable heating in your home over the winter period because you are increasingly feeling the cold. You have a problem which needs a practical solution. Considerations may be budget and portability/size of heating.

It might be that as part of your wellness plan, you like to see a homeopath every couple of months. Your need is for a natural medical approach for specific problems and as a preventative measure. Considerations may be locality, budget, gender of homeopath and support measures of the homeopath.

Factors influencing the behaviour of buyers

Culture, attitudes and beliefs are one factor that influences buying behaviour. As you grow up, you are influenced by family who teach you wrong or right. You learn about religion and culture, which helps to develop opinions, attitudes and beliefs. These factors influence your buying behaviour. Other influences include the media, those whose opinion you value, colleagues and friends who have particular experience when you come to purchase – for example, a friend who is a yoga teacher who influences your decision on what yoga mat to buy. The economic environment also has an impact on consumer behaviour; for example, do buyers have a secure job and regular income to spend? What disposable income do they have?

People's social status also impacts their behaviour. What is their role within society? Are they professionals, unemployed, teens, self-employed, special needs, young parents or retired? Clearly, being a parent affects one's buying habits depending on the age of the children. The type of job people have has an impact on the types of clothes they buy. The lifestyle of someone who earns £200,000 per year is different than someone who earns £20,000. Personality traits also have an influence on buying decisions; for example, whether the person is extrovert or introvert has an impact on the types of purchases made.

Client motivation

A potential buyer needs to be motivated in order to buy. Wellness clients want to:

- win over others by being healthier, more attractive, more fit, etc.
- live in a clean environment
- eat good food
- avoid or end pain
- have good health and live longer
- belong to a select group (who have wellness coaching)
- have an easier life
- feel secure and safe
- satisfy their curiosity about things that could affect their current lifestyle
- invest in their (wellness) future
- experience the latest and newest things in life
- solve their problems
- overcome obstacles (so they can achieve their goals)
- save time (because it will make them feel more relaxed)
- look better (because it will make them feel more attractive)
- learn something new (because it will make them feel more intelligent)
- live longer (because it will make them feel healthier)

- be comfortable (because it will make them feel relieved)

- be loved (because it will make them feel wanted)

- gain pleasure (because it will make them feel more fulfilled – they may want satisfy their appetite or sexual desires).

There are two principal ways to evaluate the motivation behind consumer purchases:

- Direction: *Direction* refers to what the client wants from a service or product. For example, if a client needs pain relief, he may like the idea that one therapist has lower fees than another…but what he really wants is fast pain relief, and he will probably pay more if he thinks the more expensive therapist can do that more effectively and quicker.

- Intensity: *Intensity* refers to whether clients' interest in a wellness service or product is compelling (or motivating) enough that they will become buyers.

MASLOW'S HIERARCHY OF NEEDS

Abraham Maslow's Hierarchy of Needs theory explains what motivates individuals to achieve. He suggests individuals' first aim is to meet basic psychological needs of hunger and thirst. When this has been met, they move up to the next stage of the hierarchy: safety needs, such as having a job, home etc. Social needs come next: for example the need to belong. Then we move up to esteem needs, such as the need for status and recognition. At the top of the hierarchy comes self-actualization which is the realization that an individual has reached their potential in life (which means something different to everyone). For more detail see Module 3.

Marketing is about meeting needs and providing benefits. Maslow's concept suggests that needs change as we travel our path towards self-actualization. For example, Tescos meet the psychological needs of hunger and thirst, while Harvey Nichols develops products for those who want their esteem needs met. Maslow's concept can be a useful tool to help understand and develop consumer needs and wants.

Information search

Let's suppose we're looking for a homeopath. Where shall we look? What budget do we set ourselves? What experience are we looking for? Potential clients like to be informed in order to reach their buying decision. Sources of information could be the Internet, personal recommendation, the local health food shop, an article or family and friends who may have been through the same thing.

Inside tip

In theory, the market for wellness coaching is almost limitless – at some time or another, everyone needs coaching. Demand is affected by the state of the economy. When the economy is buoyant, people are more likely to spend money on self-improvement services (which may be seen as a luxury and therefore a discretionary spend, unlike paying the gas bill, which is essential). When the economy weakens, people cut back on the amount of money they spend on non-essentials. For example, they might invest in a self-help publication instead of paying for a series of wellness coaching sessions. Think about whether demand for your services can weather the downturn in the economy and how else you might package your services.

EVALUATION OF DIFFERENT PURCHASE OPTIONS

So to which therapist or wellness coach do we go to? Buyers attach varying degrees of importance to each feature of a service or product. For example, homeopath Fred Smith may be more accessible, and homeopath Mary Jones may have a better fee. For us, the fee is more important than accessibility. If the decision falls between Fred or Mary, then, who shall it be? It could be that a testimonial we read on Fred's site tips the balance, and we decide to go with that homeopath.

People are now pulling variable solutions towards them, not wanting set choices presented to them. They seek individualized options rather than set presentations.

There are four typical types of buying behaviour:

- Habitual buying behaviour: The individual buys something out of habit, e.g. a health-related magazine.

- Variety-seeking buying behaviour: The individual likes to shop around and experiment with different services, products or courses.

- Complex buying behaviour: The individual purchases a high-value wellness service or product and seeks a lot of information before the purchase is made.

- Dissonance-reducing buying behaviour: The buyer is highly involved with the purchase of the product or service because the purchase is expensive or infrequent, e.g. a retreat.

Purchase decision

Through the evaluation process, buyers will reach their final decision and go through the purchase action of going online or contacting the therapist or wellness coach by email or phone.

What you are selling

Your clients aren't buying wellness coaching, homeopathy, counselling or reflexology from you. They are buying an emotional concept:

recovery of something lost, e.g. youth	fulfilment
knowledge/self-improvement	security/safety
comfort	superiority (over others)
pain relief	improved health
an easier life	lifestyle improvement
easing or resolution of a problem	a sense of achievement
more time	relaxation
confidence	increased attractiveness
increased intelligence	a sense of belonging

The client has a need for one or more of the above. How do the above needs fit in with your wellness coaching niche? Let's have a look at some examples:

- If you are selling weight-management coaching to post-natal women, your client is buying: increased attractiveness, improved health and recovery of figure.
- If you are selling IBS coaching, your client is buying: lifestyle improvement, confidence, easing or resolution of a problem, comfort, pain relief and improved health.
- If you are selling self-esteem coaching to young people, your client is buying: confidence, security/safety, lifestyle improvement, a sense of achievement, knowledge/self-improvement.

- If you are selling stress-management coaching to social workers, your client is buying: relaxation, confidence, easing/resolution of a problem, improved health and lifestyle improvement.

62 wellness ideas for wellness coaching

1. When people feel it's their idea to buy, they will be less hesitant. Tell them in your ad 'You're making a smart decision coming for wellness coaching'.

2. Promote yourself as well as your products and services. Write articles, e-books, reports, etc.

3. Show your prospects a group of testimonials that stand up for your service or product. People are more likely to agree with a group than have a different opinion.

4. Advertise in local media such as newspaper, print, TV or cable TV.

5. Speak at industry and professional events. These are highly visible and well-attended events where you can further establish your expertise. In the tradition model, you will be invited to speak at a particular location. Increasingly, you may be invited to participate as a virtual speaker, which is a high leverage opportunity to give lots of presentations to groups of prospects around the world, without leaving home.

6. Hire a marketing consultant.

7. Offer a quality product or service as an up-sell. You won't have to create a totally new product or service – just add on to your main one.

8. Make your service or product offer as 'rarely available'. People perceive things that are rare as being more valuable. You could use a limited-time offer or free bonuses.

9. As GPs become increasingly responsible for local budgets, it would be worthwhile approaching them to get wellness coaching referrals.

10. Offer a limited-time free bonus. For example, book a wellness coaching intensive before April 2 and get a free bonus!

11. Tie in your offline marketing with your website.

12. Raise your visibility. In order for your wellness business to be successful, you need to reach potential clients across multiple channels. Six ways you could do this include:

    a. offline advertising, such as Yellow Pages

    b. online advertising such as free and paid directories

    c. attending and creating PR events

    d. writing a book related to your specialisms

    e. writing articles for related websites and offline magazines and press

    f. linking your website to high traffic websites and offering a reciprocal link.

13. Offer a 30-minute wellness coaching session (call it 'micro coaching') for a reduced fee.

14. Market to existing clients. For service providers, the initial sale gives rise to the provision of further support, as satisfied clients become repeat buyers. Up-selling to existing clients produces more sales than trawling for new prospects. Four ways to up-sell:

    a. Build up a client database and send regular email and direct mail offering special promotions throughout the year.

    b. Reward your clients for doing more business with you by offering client discounts.

    c. When a client contracts with you for a specific service, you can up-sell by offering them additional services at an additional rate.

    d. If you see something that you can do to help your client be healthy or successful, share that with your client.

15. Use bundling. An effective way to increase your profits and sales is to bundle many products or services together into one package. This gives people more reasons to buy your products and services, since they perceive package deals as good value. You want all the products or services to be closely related. You could survey your customers and see what products or services they would like you to offer in the future. Look at your competition and see what products and services they're offering or not offering. Bundling can also increase your target markets which in return would give you a larger audience to sell your products and services to. Some people buy a package deal just to get one of the products. There are many sources where you can find products and services to create a package deal. You can buy them from wholesalers or drop shippers. You can buy the reproduction/resell rights to other people's products. Team-up with your competition to create a package deal. You could joint venture or offer cross-promotion deals with other businesses. You could also create your own products and services. As a service provider, you want to offer quality which is often seen through price. Rather than lowering your fees, which may be perceived as a service of less worth, add value by bundling services or products or

bundling services with products. This will increase the perceived value of what you offer in the eyes of your clients. Here are three ways you could add value:

    a. Give away free samples of a product or a mini treatment, for regular clients.

    b. Offer a yearly or biannual consultation to discuss their wellness programme at no charge and to review progress and goals.

    c. Partner with a similar (but not directly competitive) business and collaborate on a bundle to offer to clients.

16. Donate a percentage of all coaching revenue in a particular month to your favourite charity. Publicize it with a press release to the media.

17. Call your best clients and tell them about your end-of-year special created specifically for them.

18. Use buddy marketing to promote your business. For example, if you send out brochures, you could include a leaflet and/or business card of another related business who has agreed to do the same for you. This gives you the chance to reach a whole new pool of potential customers and clients.

19. Get involved in community-service activities.

20. Create workshops on wellness-related topics.

21. Offer gift certificates and e-vouchers for wellness coaching.

22. Hold a client/customer appreciation day with a special wellness coaching Q&A session or in-person lunch.

23. Design a wellness coaching calendar filled with thoughts and inspirations for every day.

24. Conduct a wellness-industry survey and publish results in your newsletter, etc.

25. Launch a new membership site or online community, free or paid, and invite subscribers and clients to join.

26. Offer all of your wellness coaching products as a bundle for one special price for a particular time period.

27. Use other people to sell your wellness-related products. In addition to selling your products yourself, look for existing mail order companies that would be willing to include your products in their catalogues, or for distributors or sales agents to take over sales chores for you. (Be sure your pricing structure allows for the fees or commissions you will have to pay on any sales that are made.)

28. Win more referrals. Past and existing clients can give referrals. So can strategic business partnerships which attract your client base. Ensure your referrers have an easy point of contact, such as your website or business card, and make sure the phone gets answered, emails get responses and you follow up on referral leads. You could offer referral fees and give something back to your referrers every time they refer a new client.

29. Become an online expert. Research active email discussion lists and online bulletin boards that are relevant to your wellness coaching market and audience. Join several and start posting expert advice to solve problems or answer questions.

30. Create a list of New Year's resolutions in your niche (e.g. 'Top 10 New Year's Resolutions for a Better Relationship') and submit it as a press release or publish as an article.

31. Find ways to differentiate. Careful differentiation is essential to successfully growing a service business. What sets your business apart from all the rest? Perhaps it's the group of services you offer or the way you excel at client satisfaction. For best results, identify the unique benefits you provide, and make them the central focus of your marketing message. Six ways you can differentiate:

    a. by providing your product/service in a way that no other business does

    b. in the quality of products you use

    c. by your track record in the industry

    d. by creating an innovative treatment programme

    e. through added value

    f. by providing excellent client service and back-up.

32. Create a list of the 12 days of wellness self-coaching – things people can do for themselves. Submit it as a press release or publish in your newsletter.

33. Write a special holiday issue of your wellness newsletter; include highlights of your year, your clients' success stories and your goals and plans for next year. Inspire your readers to take action towards personal growth!

34. Announce a contest to win a seat in the upcoming wellness coaching programme, coaching club or coaching 'gym'.

> ### Inside tip
>
> Wellness coaching clients can come from GPs, private hospitals, employers, disease management organizations, support groups, fitness centres, sports clubs, health food shops, insurance companies, herb and supplement providers, employee assistance providers, wellness companies, beauty salons, gyms, spas, therapists, health clubs and leisure centres.

35. Create an end-of-year sale on coaching books and products.

36. Create a range of useful, give-away promotional material with your logo, name and contact details such as pens, mugs, notebooks, T-shirts, etc. It's an inexpensive way to surround your prospects or clients with your branding.

37. Create a wellness retreat and invite your clients to relax and learn.

38. Partner with local spas to create a one-day wellness coaching spa retreat.

39. Offer laser-coaching sessions to the first ten people who sign up for your new 'January New Year Group Coaching Programme'.

40. Create a deck of 52 wellness inspiration cards – one for each week.

41. Create and sell a wellness coaching journal for your clients to use throughout the year.

42. Sell creative jars filled with affirmations called 'Wellness Bottles' with 'take as needed' inscriptions inside.

43. Make someone's dream come true; coach someone for free and then publicize it.

44. Start a new online or offline wellness publication and announce it to your mailing list and to the media.

45. Write a wellness-related column in your local newspaper.

46. Speaking at your local radio station on wellness.

47. Create an email newsletter to further expand your visibility within your wellness niche. This is a free way to stay in touch with your prospects on a frequent basis. Make it easy for them to forward your newsletter to others. Once you decide on the frequency of your newsletter, here are some examples of what to include in it:

a. your free monthly article

b. updates of your services and products

c. an invitation to a free tele-seminar

d. cutting edge information on a particular wellness aspect

e. the details of where you will be speaking in-person or as a virtual presenter.

48. If you have more than one niche, provide a free newsletter for each group, customizing it each time.

49. Attend networking opportunities.

50. Build strategic alliances. The goal of living in your niche is being highly visible within the industry/profession of your clients and prospects. This means selecting strategic alliance partners who will add more value and visibility to your business. In turn, you must be clear about the value and visibility you bring to your alliance partner. Think high-impact, high-visibility and win-win. Consider creating a strategic alliance with:

a. a non-competing website that your clients visit frequently or that sells to the same clients you are targeting

b. a book publisher who markets to your prospective client base

c. the organizations that serve the wellness needs of your prospective buyers

d. a publication that is read by your prospects

e. a person who is an important influencer within your wellness market

f. a non-competing email newsletter that has subscribers who are your prospects.

51. Purchase space at wellness exhibitions and tradeshows.

52. Start a blog.

53. Take your show on the road and connect with your audience who might turn into buyers. The more you share your message, the faster you accelerate in building the business. Ask yourself: Where can I speak? – How can I get my writing published? – Where can I volunteer? – Who can I call or email? – On what sites can I blog? – What gatherings can I go to?

54. Lots of coaches focus on the *what* they want to coach and try to sell that. It rarely works. Focus instead on a *who* target market, and you'll enjoy better success.

55. Use social media like Facebook, LinkedIn, etc., to get to the people.

56. Build an effective relationship with your coaching list. People do not care about how many bits of paper you have telling them how qualified you are. What people want to know is why they should listen to you. How do they know you can fix the pain they are in? The coaching is almost irrelevant; it's the result they will pay you money for. Give them something of value that will help them get rid of or ease their current problem. People will not buy high-price packages off you on a first encounter. You have to build their trust and earn the right to sell to them.

57. Productizing your coaching will help to establish your credibility. Write that free report, record a CD, write a book and self-publish it.

58. Write articles designed to position you as an expert in the eyes of your prospective of clients. The article is not designed to be a commercial about you. By sharing knowledge, insight, trends and tips your clients will remember the expertise you provide. The articles can be between 300 and 700 words long and can be used in several different formats, such as:

    a. posted on your website
    b. mentioned within an list-serve or e-zine
    c. sent to several popular related sites where your prospects might visit
    d. used as a foundation for training
    e. included as part of the script for a wellness-related DVD
    f. placed into a workbook
    g. included as part of the script for a wellness-related CD
    h. used when making a speech, etc.
    i. included in a newsletter (yours or someone else's) your buyers might read
    j. submitted to a offline publication which your target market reads
    k. included in a wellness-related CD-ROM.

59. When your articles are placed with this kind of visibility, your buyers will experience what you have to share on two levels. They might read your articles, be impressed with what you have to share and contact you for more information. On a deeper level, the people reading your articles will perceive you to be an expert within your field, which is why your article was selected over other authors and wellness coaches.

60. Joining key industry or professional committees will increase your credibility and allow you to further leverage the visibility of your wellness products and services. You will also be giving something back to the community.

61. Host free tele-seminars. Technology makes it quick, easy and cost-effective to host national and international tele-seminar calls for five to a hundred or more participants. Invite prospective clients to join a free monthly tele-seminar led by you. Some ideas:

    a. educate participants on the information covered in your most recent article or book

    b. coach a focus group

    c. invite participants to speak with you or a guest

    d. provide tips for how to manage a particular condition

    e. provide tips for how to increase wellness.

62. Use a free tele-seminar as a hook to a paying one.

Creating a wellness coaching marketing plan (ABC Business Consulting 2010)

A strong marketing plan means you have a clear idea of how you will get your wellness coaching in front of potential buyers. A good marketing plan:

- sets clear, realistic and measurable targets
- includes deadlines for meeting targets
- provides a budget for each marketing activity.

Step 1: Industry analysis

Start analyzing the wellness coaching industry; its current state, major players, industry changes, economic modelling forecasts and growth areas. You are gathering two types of information:

1. The first is primary information that you will compile yourself or pay someone else to gather. When conducting primary research there are two types of information; exploratory and specific. Exploratory research is open-ended, helps define a specific problem and usually involves interviews where answers are solicited from a targeted group via direct mail, telemarketing or personal interviews.

2. Most information will be secondary (already compiled and organized for you) and are divided into three main categories:

a. Public, e.g. governmental departments, business section of public libraries.

b. Educational, e.g. colleges, universities, and polytechnic.

c. Commercial (could involve a subscription/association fee), e.g. research and trade associations, financial institutions, publicly traded corporations.

Step 2: Market segments

Narrow your focus to define and analyze your wellness coaching market segments. You would have begun to do this in Module 7: Niching Wellness Coaching. Niching allows you to clarify how your wellness coaching products and services apply to these different segments, including the perceived benefits which speak to that particular segment. For consumer segmentation, there are variables you can use to get an idea of your ideal buyer:

- Geographic area.
- Demographics: Age, gender, income level, marital status, religious or ethnic background, wants/needs.
- Psychographics: Buying behaviour, personality, values, spending patterns, brand consciousness, lifestyle, activities and interests.

Once you have selected a target segment, consider:

- Is the segment large enough to go after?
- How difficult will it be to reach this segment with your marketing strategies?
- Does this segment have the need and money to grow your wellness coaching business?
- Is the segment expanding? How many wellness coaches are already servicing that segment?
- Do you have the necessary skills, knowledge and expertise to service the segment?

Look at your current client base and see if there is a pattern. What characteristics do the majority have in common that you could turn into a segment? Often the most promising segments are those in which you have existing clients.

Step 3: Target markets

With your market segmentation strategy outlined, you can now narrow down your target markets, determining the niches you can effectively go after. Let's take a look at an example. Reflexologists would start by picking their target market based on geographic location, since it is more likely that their client base will come from within a ten-mile radius of their clinic. However, within that target market, you could segment even more to offer wellness coaching based on wellness needs:

- Would stressed corporate executives benefit from reflexology, which you could blend with niche wellness coaching (time management, work/life balance etc)?

- Athletes or dancers could benefit from reflexology for foot and leg circulation as well as improving energy. Could you blend reflexology with niche wellness coaching (using imagery for peak performance, etc.)?

- Considering we are an ageing population, could you blend reflexology for seniors, into which you could add niche wellness coaching (managing specific health issues, fitness and mobility, etc.)?

When defining market needs, define your products and services in terms of target market needs and focus on the buyer needs you satisfy. Determine why clients buy from you and formulate that strategy behind your market segmentation. Here is a checklist of what you need to know about potential buyers:

- ✓ Who they are: If you sell directly to individuals, find out your clients' gender, age and occupation. If you sell to the corporate sector, find out their size and type of business.

- ✓ What they do: If you sell directly to individuals, it's worth knowing their occupations and interests. If you sell to the corporate sector, it helps to have an understanding of what the employees might need in relation to wellness. Do they have any particular wellness needs which reflect their industry? For example, dancers might benefit from reflexology to stimulate foot circulation (along with the other benefits of reflexology!) and anxiety/performance coaching.

- ✓ Why they buy: If you know why clients buy a product or service, it's easier to match their needs to the benefits your business can offer.

- ✓ When they buy: If you approach a client just at the time they want to buy, you will massively increase your chances of success. For example, offer weight management in January or exam stress management at key points in the university timetable.

- ✓ How they buy: For example, some people prefer to buy from a website while others prefer a face-to-face meeting.

- ✓ How much money they have: You'll be more successful if you can match what you're offering to what you know your client can afford.

- ✓ What makes them feel good about buying: If you know what makes them tick, you can serve them in the way they prefer.

- ✓ What they expect of you: For example, if your clients expect quick service and you don't disappoint them, you stand to gain repeat business.

- ✓ What they think about you: If your clients enjoy dealing with you and are satisfied with your products or service, they're likely to buy more. And you can only tackle problems that clients have if you know what they are.

- ✓ What they think about your competitors: If you know how your clients view your competition, you stand a much better chance of staying ahead of your rivals.

Step 4: Market trends and growth rates

When you have analyzed the direction of market trends in the wellness sector from a strategic standpoint, you can project the market growth in order to identify links between buyers, income and profit. Based on this, you can get some idea of return on investment (ROI) and work out the budget required so you can finance the growth.

Step 5: Competitive analysis

Now you need to look at your competition and analyze why clients might choose one wellness coach over another and why clients will buy from you instead of your competitors. The analysis needs to include:

- a comparison between your wellness products and services' variables, such as pricing, trends, quality, perceived value, reputation, product packaging, advertising, client service, target market focus, innovation, brand awareness, etc., and your competitors'

- your top four competitive strengths and weaknesses

- your top competitive gap threats

- how you can bridge your competitive gaps and in what areas your business is better than the competition. What is your positioning strategy and what are your niche areas and customization?

- an analysis of areas such as cost structure, distribution of products, trade secrets, service and product differential, etc., to determine how you can effectively protect your competitive edge and future growth.

Step 6: Pulling together your marketing strategy

You need to pull together these core components of your marketing strategy:

1. Positioning statements: Focus on the wellness coaching market's most important needs and how your products and services meet those needs. List your main competition and how your products and services are better. Once you have decided on your target market, decide how you will position yourself in it. For example, you might offer a high-quality service at a premium price, or a flexible local service at a lower rate. You might offer deluxe wellness-related products with an exclusive slant or low-price downloadable products. Whatever your strategy, you want to differentiate yourself from the competition.

2. Pricing strategy: Provide a price breakdown of your products and services, and relate your pricing determinants and strategy to your overall marketing strategy. Consider things like the sales and production cost of your products; the cost of your services; what your margins will be; discount strategies; dealer and distributor margins for products; how pricing will change over time, etc.

3. Promotion strategy: How are you going to market your wellness coaching business to future clients? How is your marketing different to your competitors'? You might want to think about: trade shows, PR, press advertising, exhibitions, retail outlets, direct mail, community events, Internet strategies, seminars, workshops and conferences. You need to consider the cost of marketing activities against expected response rates.

4. Product distribution strategy: If you sell products as part of your wellness business, how will you distribute them and what is unique in your strategy compared to your competitors'?

Step 7: Anticipating market changes

Your marketing strategy should conclude with determining the changes over the next three to five years which would impact your business. What potential changes can harm your market and bring advantage in your market? How can you prepare for these changes? A marketing strategy is organic, always developing and adjusting to market conditions, trends and changes.

Find marketing resources on the Chartered Institute of Marketing website at www.cim.co.uk.

CPD task sheet

This is your Continuing Professional Development (CPD) task sheet which summarizes key module points and offers you the opportunity to engage with tasks to deepen your learning.

Module summary

- As healthcare professionals, we need to understand consumer buying behaviour to create our marketing strategy accordingly. We need to identify what we are selling and tailor it to 'speak the marketing language' to our potential buyers.

Your task

Create your marketing plan for your wellness coaching practice.

Last Words

I hope you have enjoyed reading this book. If you would like to take your learning further, you may be interested in the Diploma in Wellness Coaching and other CPD courses that I offer for wellness professionals.

I would also like to offer you this 5 per cent discount voucher applicable to any qualification courses or business-coaching opportunities on my site. You are most welcome to visit www.wellnessprofessionalsatwork.com to find out more.

References

Module 1

BCC Research (2009) 'Anti-aging products and services: The global market.' Available at www.bccresearch.com/report/anti-aging-products-services-hlc060a.html, accessed on 9 June 2011.

Beveridge, W. (1942) *Social Insurance and Allied Services*. London: BBC. Available at http://news.bbc.co.uk/1/shared/bsp/hi/pdfs/19_07_05_beveridge.pdf, accessed on 6 December 2010.

Bupa (undated a) *Health Coaching*. Available at www.bupa.co.uk/healthcare-providers/bupa-health-dialog/products-and-solutions/clinical-claims-management-1, accessed on 1 December 2010.

Bupa (undated b) *Introducing a New Collaborative Care Model for the UK's NHS*. Available at http://bupa.com/healthcare/healthcare-affordability/nhs-collaborative-care-model, accessed on 1 December 2010.

Bupa (undated c) *Pioneering Health Coaching Services in Spain and France*. Available at bupa.com/healthcare/informed-patient-decisions/health-coaching-services, accessed on 1 December 2010.

CBC News (2010) 'Artificial pancreas tested in kids with diabetes.' Available at www.cbc.ca/news/health/story/2010/02/05/artificial-pancreas.html, accessed on 21 April 2011.

eHealthNews (2010) 'Orkney Health and Care launches telehealth initiative to improve care for patients with long-term conditions.' Available at http://ehealthnews.eu/tunstall/2242-orkney-health-and-care-launches-telehealth-initiative-to-improve-care-for-patients-with-long-term-conditions, accessed on 2 December 2010.

Fenton, S. (2009) 'UAE health market worth $12bn by 2015.' Available at www.ameinfo.com/185709.html, accessed on 1 December 2010.

Furlong, M. (2007) *Turning Silver into Gold: How to Profit in the New Boomer Marketplace*. Upper Saddle River, NJ: Financial Times Press.

Imperial College Healthcare NHS Trust (2011) 'How healthcare has changed.' Available at www.imperial.nhs.uk/nhs60/past60years/how_healthcare_has_changed/index.htm, accessed on 25 May 2011.

Institute of Medicine (2005) *Complementary and Alternative Medicine in the United States*. Available at http://iom.edu/Reports/2005/Complementary-and-Alternative-Medicine-in-the-United-States.aspx, accessed on 25 May 2011.

Izzard, J. (2007) 'Sun, sightseeing and plastic surgery.' *BBC News*. Available at http://news.bbc.co.uk/1/hi/uk/6933490.stm, accessed on 30 May 2011.

MarketsandMarkets (2010) 'Global home healthcare market worth US$159.6 billion by 2014.' Available at http://marketsandmarkets.com/PressReleases/home-health-care-market.asp, accessed on 1 December 2010.

Medical News Today (2009) 'New study shows coaching to patient activation levels improves disease management outcomes.' Available at www.medicalnewstoday.com/articles/153469.php, accessed on 1 December 2010.

Melko, C., Terry, P., Camp, K., Min, X. and Healey, M. (2010) 'Diabetes health coaching improves medication adherence: A pilot study.' *American Journal of Lifestyle Medicine 4*, 2, 187–194.

National Center for Complementary and Alternative Medicine (NCCAM) (2010) *What is Complementary and Alternative Medicine?* Available at http://nccam.nih.gov/health/whatiscam, accessed on 1 December 2010.

NHS West Essex (2009) *Improving your Health with Community Health Coaches.* Available at www.westessexpct.nhs.uk/ournews/news2009item.php?id=125, accessed on 1 December 2010.

Palmer, S., Tubbs, I. and Whybrow, A. (2003) 'Health coaching to facilitate the promotion of healthy behaviour and achievement of health-related goals.' *International Journal of Health Promotion and Education 41*, 3, 91–93.

Stratmann, L. (2009) 'Reduction in hospitalization through a whole patient health coaching program.' *International Journal of Integrated Care 9*, Annual Conference Supplement.

The Cochrane Collaboration (2010) Cochrane Complementary Medicine Field Bursary Scheme. Available at www.cochrane.org/policy-manual/251-cochrane-complementary-medicine-field-bursary-scheme, accessed on 25 May 2011.

The Hartman Group (2010) *Reimagining Health and Wellness: Lifestyle and Trends Report 2010.* Available at http://hartman-group.com/publications/reports/reimagining-health-wellness-lifestyle-and-trends-report-2010, accessed on 2 December 2010.

Trend Hunter Magazine (2009a) 'Anti-ageing spa pods.' Available at www.trendhunter.com/trends/youth-and-health-rejuvenation-oxygen-baths-prevent-cancer-and-make-you-look, accessed on 2 December 2010.

Trend Hunter Magazine (2009b) 'Nurse robots.' Available at www.trendhunter.com/trends/nursing-robots-riba, accessed on 2 December 2010.

Trend Hunter Magazine (2009c) 'Stick-on stamina.' Available at www.trendhunter.com/trends/software-for-the-human-body, accessed on 2 December 2010.

Trend Hunter Magazine (2009d) 'Virtual health coaches.' Available at www.trendhunter.com/trends/virtual-personal-trainer-brauns-coach-nurse-for-the-price-of-one, accessed on 2 December 2010.

Trend Hunter Magazine (2010) 'DIY healthcare.' Available at www.trendhunter.com/tv/diy-healthcare-sprint-firsts-in-futuristic-medical-technology, accessed on 2 December 2010.

United Nations (2009) 'World population to exceed 9 billion by 2050.' Available at www.un.org/esa/population/publications/wpp2008/pressrelease.pdf, accessed on 26 May 2011.

Vale, M., Jelinek, M., Best, J. and Dart, A. (2003) 'Coaching patients On Achieving Cardiovascular Health (COACH): A multicenter randomized trial in patients with coronary heart disease.' *Archives of Internal Medicine 163*, 2775–2783.

What's Next (2011) 'Top trends in healthcare, medicine and pharmaceuticals.' Available at http://nowandnext.com/?action=top_trend/list_trends&sectorId=10, accessed on 2 December 2010.

Module 2

Ader, R. and Cohen, N. (1975) 'Behaviourally conditioned immunosupression.' *Psychosomatic Medicine 37*, 4, 333–340.

Ader, R., Felten, D.L. and Cohen, N. (2006) *Psychoneuroimmunology.* Burlington, MA: Academic Press.

American Institute of Stress (2010) 'America's No.1 Health Problem.' Available at www.stress.org/americas.htm, accessed on 6 December 2010.

Beard, G. (1884) *Practical Treatise on Nervous Exhaustion (Neurasthenia).* New York: Treat.

Benson, H. (1975) *The Relaxation Response.* New York: Morrow.

Benson, H., Beary, J.F. and Carol, M.P. (1974) 'The Relaxation Response.' *Psychiatry 37*, 1, 37–46.

Birk, L. (ed.) (1973) *Biofeedback: Behavioural Medicine.* New York: Grune and Stratton.

British Society of Integrated Medicine (2008) 'Our definition of integrated medicine.' Available at http://bsim.org.uk, accessed on 6 December 2010.

Cabot, R.C. (1909) *Social Service and the Art of Healing.* New York: Moffat, Yard, and Company.

Cannon, W.B. (1915) *Bodily Changes in Pain, Hunger, Fear and Rage: An Account of Recent Researches into the Function of Emotional Excitement.* New York: D. Appleton and Co.

Cannon, W.B. (1932) *The Wisdom of the Body.* New York: Norton.

Dunn, L.H. (1961) *High Level Wellness.* Arlington, VA: Beatty Press.

Engel, G.L. (1977) 'The need for a New Medical Model: A challenge for biomedicine.' *Science 196,* 129–126.

Faculty of Integrated Medicine (2010) 'What is integrative medicine?' Available at http://integrativemedicine.uk.com/what_is_im.php, accessed on 6 December 2010.

Hales, D. (2003) *An Invitation to Health.* Belmont, CA: Wadsworth/Thomson Learning.

Hettler, B. (1976) 'Six dimensions of wellness model.' *National Wellness Institute.* Available at www.nationalwellness.org/pdf/SixDimensionsFactSheet.pdf, accessed on 6 June 2011.

Holmes, O.W. (1860) 'Current and Counter-currents in Medical Science.' In M. Stinson (ed.) (2009) *Medical Essays.* Chicago, IL: SBI, Inc.

Holmes, T.H. and Rahe, R.H. (1967) 'The social readjustment rating scale.' *Journal of Psychosomatic Research 11,* 213–218.

Jacobson, E. (1938) *Progressive Relaxation.* Chicago, IL: University of Chicago Press.

Kiecolt-Glaser, J.K., McGuire, L., Robles, T.F. and Glaser, R. (2002) 'Psychoneuroimmunology: Psychological influences on immune function and health.' *Journal of Consulting and Clinical Psychology 70,* 3, 537–547. Available at http://pni.osumc.edu/KG%20Publications%20%28pdf%29/150.pdf, accessed on 1 June 2011.

Medical Wellness Association (2003) 'Defining medical wellness.' Available at http://medicalwellnessassociation.com/articles/defining_medical_wellness.htm, accessed on 6 December 2010.

Miller, C. (2004) *Nursing for Wellness in Older Adults.* New York: Lippincott, Williams, Wilkins.

Miller, N.E. (1969) 'Learning of visceral and glandular responses.' *Science 163,* 434–445.

National Center for Complementary and Alternative Medicine (NCCAM) (2010) 'What is complementary and alternative medicine?' Available at http://nccam.nih.gov/health/whatiscam, accessed on 21 April 2010.

O'Donnell (1989) 'Definition of health promotion.' *American Journal of Health Promotion 3,* 3, 5.

Ornish, D. (1999) *Love and Survival.* New York: Harper Paperbacks.

Pelletier, K. (1977) *Mind as Healer, Mind as Slayer.* New York: Delta.

Pert, C.B., Ruff, M.R., Weber, R.J. and Herkenham, M. (1985) 'Neuropeptides and their receptors: A psychosomatic network.' *Journal of Immunology 135,* 820s–826s.

Pilates, J. (1998/1934) *Your Health.* New York: Presentation Dynamics.

Pilates, J.H. and Miller, W.J. (1998/1945) *Pilates' Return to Life Through Contrology.* New York: Presentation Dynamics.

Pilzer, P.Z. (2007) *The New Wellness Revolution: How to Make a Fortune in the Next Trillion Dollar Industry.* New York: John Wiley and Sons.

Rochester Review (1997) 'The mind-body connection: Granny was right, after all.' University of Rochester, Rochester. Available at http://rochester.edu/pr/Review/V59N3/feature2.html, accessed on 6 December 2010.

Rogers, C. (1951) *Client-centred Therapy: Its Current Practice, Implications and Theory.* London: Constable.

Ruff, M., Schiffmann, E., Terranova, V. and Pert, C. (1985) 'Neuropeptides are chemoattractants for human tumor cells and monocytes: A possible mechanism for metastasis.' *Clinical Immunology and Immunopathology 37*, 3, 387–396.

Selye, H. (1936) 'A syndrome produced by diverse nocuous agents.' *Nature 138*, 32. Available at http://neuro.psychiatryonline.org/cgi/content/full/10/2/230a, accessed on 21 April 2010.

Selye, H. (1956) *The Stress of Life*. New York: McGraw-Hill.

Selye, H. (1973) 'The evolution of the stress concept.' *American Scientist 61*, 692–699.

Selye, H. (1974) *Stress without Distress*. Philadelphia, PA: J.B. Lippincott Co.

Siegelman, E. (1983) *Personal Risk: Mastering Change in Love and Work*. New York: Harper and Row.

Snyderman, R. and Weil, A.T. (2002) 'Integrative medicine: Bringing medicine back to its roots.' *Archives of Internal Medicine 162*, 4, 395–397.

Solomon, G.F. and Moos, R.H. (1964) 'Emotions, immunity, and disease: A speculative theoretical integration.' *Archives of General Psychiatry 11*, 657–674.

Spiegel, D. (2010) *Stanford School of Medicine Centre on Stress and Health*. Available at http://stresshealthcenter.stanford.edu, accessed on 6 December 2010.

Toffler, A. (1970) *Future Shock*. New York: Random House

Wein, H. (2009) 'Stress and disease: New perspectives.' *Stress, Anxiety and Depression Resource Center*. Article syndicated from National Institute of Health. Available at www.stress-anxiety-depression.org/stress/disease.html, accessed on 1 June 2011.

Wolff, H.G. (1953) *Stress and Disease*. Springfield, IL: Charles C. Thomas.

World Health Organization (1948) 'WHO definition of health.' Available at http://who.int/about/definition/en/print.html, accessed on 6 December 2010.

World Health Organization (1986) *Ottawa Charter for Health Promotion*. Available at http://who.int/hpr/NPH/docs/ottawa_charter_hp.pdf, accessed on 6 December 2010.

Module 3

Adams, K. (1998) *The Way of the Journal: A Journey Therapy Workbook for Healing*. Towson, MD: Sidran Press.

Bruce, R. (1998) 'Strange but true: Improve your health through journaling.' *Self-help Magazine*. Available at www.selfhelpmagazine.com/article/node/442, accessed on 6 December 2010.

Downey, M. (2003) *Effective Coaching*. London: Texere Publishing.

Fleming, N.D. and Mills, C. (1992) 'Not another inventory, rather a catalyst for reflection.' *To Improve the Academy 11*, 137–155.

Gregorc, A.F. (1984) *Development, Technical, and Administration Manual*. Columbia, CT: Gregorc Associates.

Honey, P. and Mumford, A. (1982) *The Manual of Learning Styles*. Maidenhead: Peter Honey Publications.

Honey, P. and Mumford, A. (1983) *Using Your Learning Styles*. Maidenhead: Peter Honey Publications.

International Coach Federation (2010) 'Core competencies.' Available at www.coachfederation.org/icfcredentials/core-competencies, accessed on 6 December 2010.

Kolb, D. (1984) *Experiential Learning: Experience as the Source of Learning and Development*. Englewood Cliffs, NJ: Prentice-Hall.

Maslow, A. (1943) 'A theory of human motivation.' *Psychological Review 50*, 370–396. Available at http://psychclassics.yorku.ca/Maslow/motivation.htm, accessed on 7 December 2010.

Maslow, A. (1954) *Motivation and Personality*. New York: HarperCollins.

McLeod, A. and Thomas, W. (2010) *Performance Coaching Toolkit*. Maidenhead: Open University Press.

Miller, W.R. (1983) 'Motivational interviewing with problem drinkers.' *Behavioural Psychotherapy 11*, 147–172.

Progoff, I. (1992) *At a Journal Workshop: Writing to Access the Power of the Unconscious and Evoke Creative Ability*. Los Angeles, CA: Tarcher.

Rowe, A.J. and Mason, R.O. (1987) *Managing with Style: A Guide to Understanding, Assessing and Improving Decision-Making*. San Francisco, CA: Jossey-Bass Management Series.

Whitmore, J. (2009) *Coaching for Performance: GROWing People, Performance and Purpose*. London: Nicholas Brealey Publishing.

Module 4

Lindahl, K. (2009) 'The sacred art of listening.' Parliament of the World's Religions, 8 December 2009. Available at www.sacredlistening.com/CWPR%20Handout%20Listening%20Background. pdf, accessed on 6 June 2011.

Module 5

Abrams, M. (2011) 'REBT.' *The Albert Ellis Site*. Available at www.rebt.ws/REBT%20explained.htm, accessed on 6 June 2011.

Beck, A. (1975) *Cognitive Therapy and the Emotional Disorders*. Madison, CT: International Universities Press.

Beck, J.S. (1995) *Cognitive Therapy: Basics and Beyond*. New York: The Guilford Press.

Beutler, L.E., Moleiro, C. and Talebi, H. (2002) 'Resistance in psychotherapy: What conclusions are supported by research.' *Journal of Clinical Psychology 58*, 2, 207–217.

Ellis, A. (1957) 'Rational psychotherapy and individual psychology.' *Journal of Individual Psychology 13*, 38–44.

Ellis, A. (1962) *Reason and Emotion in Psychotherapy*. Secaucus, NJ: Citadel.

Ellis, A. and Dryden, W. (2007) *The Practice of Rational Emotive Behaviour Therapy*. New York: Springer Publishing.

Neenan, M. and Dryden, W. (2000) *Essential Rational Emotive Behaviour Therapy*. London: Whurr.

Palmer, S. (1997) 'Self-acceptance: Concept, techniques and interventions.' *The Rational Emotive Behaviour Therapist 4*, 2, 4–30.

Palmer, S. and Dryden, W. (2005) *Counselling for Stress Problems*. London: Sage Publications.

Sperry, R.W., Hubel, D.H. and Wiesel, T.N. (1981) 'Some effects of disconnecting the cerebral hemispheres.' Nobel Lecture. Available at http://nobelprize.org/nobel_prizes/medicine/laureates/1981/sperry-lectrure.html, accessed on 16 May 2011.

Wasik, B. (1984) *Teaching Parents Effective Problem Solving: A Handbook for Professionals*. Unpublished manuscript. Chapel Hill, NC: University of North Carolina.

Wolpe, J. (1969) *The Practice of Behavioural Therapy*. New York: Pergamon Press.

Module 6

Association for Applied Psychophysiology and Biofeedback (2008) 'What is biofeedback?' Available at http://aapb.org, accessed on 2 December 2010.

Association of Humanistic Psychology Practitioners (2010) *UKAHPP Core Beliefs Statement*. Available at http://ahpp.org/about/core.htm, accessed on 2 December 2010.

British Association for Applied Nutrition and Nutritional Therapy (2011) 'Understanding the differences between nutrition health professionals: "Optimum nutrition"'. Briefing note: Optimum Nutrition 03/06. Available at www.bant.org.uk/bant/jsp/briefingNote0306.faces, accessed on 2 December 2010.

British Autogenic Society (2007) 'Clinical applications of AT.' Available at www.autogenic-therapy. org.uk/0001/whatisat-00.htm, accessed at 6 December 2010.

British Society for Ecologicial Medicine (2009) 'Ecological medicine.' Available at www.ecomed.org. uk/about-the-society/ecological-medicine, accessed on 6 December 2010.

Craig, G. (undated) *The EFT Manual* (6th edition). Available at www.spiritual-web.com/downloads/ eftmanual.pdf, accessed on 1 June 2011.

Institute for Solution-Focused Therapy (2010) 'What is solution-focused therapy?' Available at www.solutionfocused.net/solutionfocusedtherapy.html, accessed on 6 December 2010.

Jacobson, E. (1938) *Progressive Relaxation*. Chicago, IL: University of Chicago Press.

Luthe, W. and Schultz, J.H. (1969) *Autogenic Therapy*. New York: Grune and Stratton Inc. (Republished in 2001 by The British Autogenic Society.)

Mindful Living Programs (2010) 'What is mindfulness-based stress reduction?' Available at www. mindfullivingprograms.com/whatMBSR.php, accessed on 6 December 2010.

National Center for Complementary and Alternative Medicine (2010) 'Meditation: An introduction.' Available at http://nccam.nih.gov/health/meditation/overview.htm, accessed on 6 December 2010.

Neenan, M. and Dryden, W. (1999) *Rational Emotive Behaviour Therapy: Advances in Theory and Practice*. London: Whurr. Available at http://rebt.org/professionals/prof_articles/reflections.pdf, accessed on 6 December 2010.

Palmer, S. (2010) 'A multimodal approach to stress management and counselling.' Available at www. managingstress.com/articles/webpage3.htm, accessed on 6 December 2010.

Perls, F., Hefferline, R. and Goodman, P. (1951) *Gestalt Therapy: Excitement and Growth in the Human Personality*. New York: Julian.

Salovey, P. and Mayer, J. (1990) 'Emotional intelligence.' *Imagination, Cognition and Personality 9*, 3, 185–211.

Seligman, M.E.P. and Csikszentmihalyi, M. (2000) 'Positive psychology: An introduction.' *American Psychologist 55*, 1, 5–14.

Stewart, I. and Joines, V. (1987) *TA Today: A New Introduction to Transactional Analysis*. Nottingham: Lifespace Publishing.

Tosey, P. and Mathison, J. (2006) 'Introducing Neuro-Linguistic Programming.' Available at www. som.surrey.ac.uk/NLP/Resources/IntroducingNLP.pdf, accessed on 1 June 2011.

Module 7

Ries, L. and Ries, A. (1998) *The 22 Immutable Laws of Branding: How to Build a Product or Service into a World-class Brand*. New York: HarperCollins.

Module 9

ABC Business Consulting (2010) 'Developing, writing and implementing a winning marketing plan.' Available at www.businessconsultingabc.com/resources/Developing$2C+Writing+and+Impleme nting+A+Winning+Marketing+Plan.pdf, accessed on 13 June 2011.

Further Reading

Module 1

Kumar, R. (2009) *Global Trends in Health and Medical Tourism*. New Delhi: SBS Publishers.

Nolen, L.A. (2010) *The Health and Wellness Insider's Guide to Durable Trends, Fleeting Fads and Innovative Ideas*. Dallas, TX: Wellness Business Forum.

Pilzer, P.Z. (2007) *The New Wellness Revolution: How to Make a Fortune in the Next Trillion Dollar Industry*. Hoboken, NJ: John Wiley and Sons.

Module 2

Association for Coaching and Passmore, J. (ed.) (2010) *Excellence in Coaching: The Industry Guide*. London: Kogan Page.

Atkinson, M. (2007) *The Mind Body Bible*. London: Piatkus.

Greener, M. (2003) *The Which? Guide to Managing Stress*. London: Which Books.

Maté, G. (2003) *When the Body Says No: Understanding the Stress Disease Connection*. Hoboken, NJ: John Wiley and Sons.

Pert, C.B. (1997) *Molecules of* Emotion. London: Pocket Books.

Proto, L. (1990) *Self Healing: How to Use Your Mind to Heal Your Body*. London: Piatkus.

Sarno, J. (1998) *The Mindbody Prescription*. New York: Warner Books.

Shapiro, D. (1990) *The BodyMind Workbook*. Wellingborough: Thorsons.

Shapiro, D. (2007) *Your Body Speaks Your Mind*. London: Piatkus.

Travis, J. and Ryan, R.S. (2004) *The Wellness Workbook* (3rd edition). New York: Celestial Arts.

Module 3

Arloski, M. (2007) *Wellness Coaching for Lasting Lifestyle Changes*. Duluth, MN: Whole Person Associates.

Maslow, A.H and Frager, R. (1987) *Motivation and Personality*. Hong Kong: Longman Asia Ltd.

Williams, P. and Davis, D. (2007) *Therapist as Life Coach*. New York: W. W. Norton and Company.

Module 4

McMahon, G. and Archer, A. (2010) *101 Coaching Strategies and Techniques*. Hove: Routledge.

Memford, J. (2007) *Life Coaching for Dummies*. Chichester: John Wiley and Sons.

Nelson-Jones, R. (2006) *Human Relationship Skills: Coaching and Self-coaching* by Richard. Hove: Routledge.

Starr, J. (2008) *The Coaching Manual*. Harlow: Pearson Education Ltd.

Module 5

Dryden, W. (2011) *Dealing with Clients' Emotional Problems in Life Coaching: A Rational-emotive and Cognitive Behaviour Therapy Approach*. Hove: Routledge.

Neenan, M. and Palmer, S. (2011) *Cognitive Behavioural Coaching in Action: An Evidence Based Approach*. Hove: Routledge.

Whitten, H. (2009) *Cognitive Behavioural Coaching Techniques for Dummies*. Chichester: John Wiley and Sons.

Module 6

Batcheller, L.J. (2001) *Journey to Health: Writing Your Way to Physical, Emotional and Spiritual Well-being*. Lincoln, NE: iUniverse.

Biswas-Diener, R. (2010) *Practicing Positive Psychology Coaching: Assessment, Activities and Strategies for Success*. Hoboken, NJ: John Wiley and Sons.

Butler, G. (2008) *Overcoming Social Anxiety and Shyness: A Self-help Guide Using Cognitive Behavioural Techniques*. New York: Basic Books.

Capacchione, L. (2001) *The Creative Journal: The Art of Finding Yourself*. Pompton Plains, NJ: New Page Books.

Clarkson, P. (2004) *Gestalt Counselling in Action* (3rd edition). London: Sage.

Davies, W. (2009) *Overcoming Anger and Irritability: A Self-help Guide Using Cognitive Behavioural Techniques* London: Constable and Robinson.

Davis, M., Robbins Eshelman, E. and McKay, M. (2008) *Relaxation and Stress Reduction Workbook* (6th edition). Oakland, CA: New Harbinger Publications.

Epstein, G. (1997) *Healing Visualizations*. New York: Bantam Doubleday Dell Publishing Group.

Espie, C. (2006) *Overcoming Insomnia and Sleep Problems: A Self-help Guide Using Cognitive Behavioral Techniques*. London: Constable and Robinson.

Fanning, P. (1988) *Visualization for Change*. Oakland, CA: New Harbinger Publications.

Fennell, M. (1999) *Overcoming Low Self Esteem: A Self-help Guide Using Cognitive Behavioural Techniques*. London: Constable and Robinson.

Gauntlett-Gilbert, J. and Grace, C. (2009) *Overcoming Weight Problems*. London: Constable and Robinson.

Kabat-Zinn, J. (1994) *Wherever You Go, There You Are: Mindfulness Meditation in Everyday Life*. New York: Hyperion.

Kinsella, P. (2007) *Cognitive Behavioural Therapy for Chronic Fatigue Syndrome*. Hove: Routledge.

Lusk, J.T. (ed.) (1992) *30 Scripts for Relaxation Imagery and Inner Healing*. Duluth, MN: Whole Person Associates.

Naparstek, B. (1994) *Staying Well with Guided Imagery*. New York: Warner Books.

O'Connor, J. and Lages, A. (2004) *Coaching with NLP: How to be a Master Coach*. London: Element.

Palmer, S. and Dryden, W. (1994) *Counselling for Stress Problems*. London: Sage.

Perkins, K.A., Conklin, C.A. and Levine, M.D. (2008) *Cognitive Behavioral Therapy for Smoking Cessation*. New York: Taylor and Francis Group.

Quest, P. (2002) *Reiki for Life: The Essential Guide to Reiki Practice*. London: Piatkus.

Scheffer, M. (2001) *The Encyclopaedia of Bach Flower Therapy*. Rochester, VT: Healing Arts Press.

Thorn, B. (2004) *Cognitive Therapy for Chronic Pain*. New York: Guilford Press.

White, C.A. (2001) *Cognitive Behaviour Therapy for Chronic Medical Conditions*. Chichester: John Wiley and Sons.

Widdowson, M. (2009) *Transactional Analysis: 100 Key Points*. Hove: Routledge.

Module 7

Thornton, C. (2010) *Group and Team Coaching*. Hove: Routledge.

Kelley, L. (2011) *How to Become a Virtual Coach (Success Motivation Coaching)*. (Self-published)

Module 8

Burkholder, P. (2007) *Start Your Own Day Spa and More: Destinaton Spa, Medical Spa, Yoga Centre, Spiritual Spa*. London: Entrepreneur Press.

McNamara, H. (2007) *Niche Marketing for Coaches: A Practical Handbook for Building a Life Coaching, Executive Coaching or Business Coaching Practice*. London: Thorogood.

Smith, M. and Puczko, L. (2009) *Health and Wellness Tourism*. Oxford: Butterworth-Heinemann.

Weede, T. (2008) *Start Your Own Personal Training Business: Your Step-By-Step Guide to Success*. California: Entrepreneur Press.

Module 9

Brown-Volkman, D. (2003) *Four Steps to Building a Profitable Coaching Practice: A Complete Marketing Resource Guide for Coaches*. Lincoln, NE: iUniverse.

Good, S. (2009) *Creative Marketing Tools for Coaches*. New York: Good Life Press.

Martin, N.A. (2009) *The Marketing Handbook for Sports and Fitness Professionals*. London: A&C Black.

Rogers, J. (2006) *Developing a Coaching Business*. Maidenhead: Open University Press.

Thomas, R.K. (2008) *Health Services Marketing: A Practitioner's Guide*. New York: Springer.

Subject Index

Note: page references to figures, tables and forms are italicized.

3-D coaching 83

ABC model 137–8, *138*
ABCDE sequence of emotional management 141–2
acceptance coaching 83
accommodator learning style 75
accountability 72–3, 177–8
action planning 156
    action plan sheet *126*
    and decision-making 175–7
    designing the actions 71–2
    example action plan *157*
    see also planning
activating events 137, *138*, 166
active listening 69–70, 113–16
addiction recovery coaching 211
advanced coaching 84
ageing 12, 15, 17, 22
    as niche market idea 208, 212
    spa pods for 20
Airload mobile phone 20
analytical coping strategy 91
anti-ageing *see* ageing
articles 218, 250
assertive behaviour coaching 57
assimilator learning style 75
AT (autogenic training) 182
attraction coaching 83
auditory learners 74
awareness 63, 71

'Baby Boomers' 15
beauty coaching 209
Beck's common cognitive errors *146*
beginner's guides 233
behavioural coping strategy 91
behavioural experiments 171–2
behaviours
    changing associations to 88
    consumer buying 239–43
    cost-benefit analysis of 166
    dealing with revelations of unlawful 129–30
    links between emotions and thoughts *144*
    in relation to change 90–1
beliefs
    belief continuum 164
    challenging and reframing 163

cost-benefit analysis of 166
irrational 137, *138*, 157–9, *162*
    uncovering 161–2
bibliotherapy 171
bigger thinking 83
biofeedback 48, 180–1
Biofeedback StressWatch 20
biosimulations 23
block removal coaching 84
Body Check Ball 20
body language 108–11
booklets 218
boundaries 56–7
brain
    and creativity 149–50, *149*, *150*
    effects of serotonin in 151
    physiology 48, 49
Braun's Clever Care Medical Coach 21
breast cancer 18, 53, 62, 92, 191
breathing techniques 151–2, 183
bundling 245–6
Bupa 25
business expansion ideas 213–20
    see also niche markets
business networking 96
businesses, healthy 21

CAM (complementary and alternative medicines)
    as business expansion idea 216
    and conventional perceptions 32–3
    definitions and therapy types 17–18
    integration with wellness coaching 46
    relation to integrated healthcare 29–30
cardiovascular health 27, 53
cathartic writing 93
CBC (cognitive behavioural coaching)
    choices and consequences 149–52, *150*
    cognitive behavioural flow chart *135*
    decision-making and action planning 175–7
    defining 135–6
    eight-step process to using 139–43
    evaluation 178

exploring and challenging faulty thinking 157–75, *162*, *163*, *168–70*
    goal selection 152–7, *153*, *154*, *157*
    implementation 177–8
    problem identification 148
    problem-solving sequences *139–43*
    recommendations for further training in 134, 181–2
    responses to situations *136*
    setting the scene for 144–7, *146*
CDs 219, 236–7
change management
    of associations to behaviour 88
    change and stress 51–2
    helping clients with 56
    importance of 89–94
    integrating lifestyle changes 39–40
Change4Life advertising campaign 16
children coaching 202–3
chronic conditions
    living with 44–5
    as niche market idea 204–5
client-centred therapy 40–1
client mindsets *see* mindsets
client motivation *see* motivation
client-related networks 95
client responsibility *see* responsibility
clients
    coaching and supporting 55–63, 94
    developing rapport with 58, 116–19
    ending relationship with 132
    establishing readiness for coaching 42, 145–7
    establishing trust and intimacy with 69
    marketing to existing 245
    negotiating tasks with 147, 176–7
    resistance of 159–63
    revealing unlawful behaviour 129–30
    skills practice 132
    tools for use with 164–72
    unengaged 129
co-creation 42–3, 69, 122–3

COACH (Coaching patients On Achieving Cardiovascular Health) 27
coaching *see* wellness coaching
cognitive behavioural coaching *see* CBC
cognitive errors 145, *146*
cognitive wellness 36
coherent niche 202
collapsed-coping statement 171
communication, effective 69–70
communication skills 186
community health coaches 16, 27
community health coaching 206–7
compassion 55–6
competitive analysis 254
complementary and alternative medicines *see* CAM
conceptual coping strategy 91
conditioning 62
conditions, specific and chronic 44–5, 204–5
confidence, lack of 130
constructive feedback 119, *120*
consultancy 214–15
consumer buying behaviour 239–43
consumer spending 21–2
contracting 166
converger learning style 75
coping strategies 91–2
corporate wellness 205
cost-benefit analysis 166
counselling
    balance with wellness coaching 41–2, 45, 128–9
    principles 67
courses 219
CPD (Continuing Professional Development) task sheets 28, 64–5, 97, 133, 179, 194, 222, 238, 256
CPD-related networks 95
creativity
    and the brain 149–50, *150*
    creative approaches 58
    creative flow chart *149*
    creative psyche 150–2
'credit records' 165
cue exposure 166
cultural differences 130
curative approach 43
customized treatments 23

de-catastrophizing continuum 171
decision-making
    and action planning 175–7
    styles of 91–2
deep coaching 83
demanding clients 61
depression 23, 90
deserted-island technique 171
diabetes studies and trials 23, 25–6
dialogue 94
differentiation 247
directive coping strategy 91

displacement 56
distinction coaching 83
distress, reduction of 172–5
diverger learning style 75
DIY healthcare 14–15
DM (disease management) 26–7
DuoFertility monitor 21
DVDs 219, 236
dying 45

e-books 220, 234–5
e-coaching 232
e-zines 218
eclecticism 30, *31*
EFT (emotional freedom technique) 191
elaboration questions 112–13
ELT (experiential learning theory) 75
emotional intelligence 188
emotional management, sequence of 141–2
emotional shifts 110–11
emotional wellness 36
emotions
    in ABC model 137–8, *138*
    dealing with clients' 129
    links between thoughts and behaviours *144*
    links with illness 49–50
    in STEPPA coaching model 79
employee wellness 205
environmental wellness 38–9, 190
ergonomics coaching 211
ethical guidelines 68
ethics 23
ethnic communities coaching 213
evaluation
    of CBC 178
    of workshops 227
events, activating 137, *138*, 166
exergaming 21
expectations of client 60, 61, 63, 121
expert interviews 234
expression
    body, as means of 108–9
    symbolic 62
    of vulnerability 61
external organ helpers 23
extreme self-care coaching 82, 83

face, as means of expression 108–9
face-to-face coaching 223–4
failure, fear of 86, 154–5
faith 57–8
faulty thinking *see* thinking, faulty
fear
    clients' 62
    of failure 86, 154–5
    of impacting relationships 87
    of imperfection 85–6
    of rejection 87–8
    of success 87
feedback 119, *120*
feeling questions 112

feelings, reflecting 115
fight-or-flight response 48, 50–1, 52
fitness-based coaching 208, 209–10
Fleming's VAK/VARK model of learning 74, 118
flower remedies 184
food industry effects on services and products *14*
food journal 93
forgiveness 61
France, Bupa in 25

gender 212
German control study on whole-patient health coaching 24–5
Gestalt therapy 188
gestures, as means of expression 110
global thinking 164
goal setting 72, 76–7, 123–4, 152–7
Golden Boomer generation 15, 213
grace coaching 83
graded task performance 165
Gregorc's model of learning 73–4
grieving 62
group coaching 225–7
GROW model 76–7

habits
    control of 167
    cost-benefit analysis of 166
Hartman Group 21–2
health
    defining 31–2
    role of stress on 52–4
health coaching models 24–7, 82
health markets 12–13
health promotion 214
health sector sales 15
healthcare
    changing face of 16–20
    DIY 14–15
    mindsets 32–3
    trends 20–4
    see also integrated healthcare
Hibbard, J. 26
hierarchy of needs concept 84, 241
holidays 210, 216–17
home health services 15, 19–20
Honey and Mumford Learning Styles Questionnaire 76
hope 57–8
humanistic psychology 183–4

image coaching 204
imagery 168, *168–70*, 184–5
immune systems 48, 49–50, 52–3
imperfection, fear of 85–6
implementation of CBC 177–8
industry analysis 251–2
information
    availability 12
    for industry analysis 251–2
    online 21
    products 218–20, 233–8
    searching 241

informed clients 58–9
innovation coaching 83
integrated healthcare
  challenges 33
  with client mindsets 54–63, 128
  defining 29–30
  with mindbody 46–54
  and the wellness coach 40–5
  and wellness coaching 45–6,
    63–4, 64
integrity coaching 84
interactive text coaching 232
intermediate coaching 83
internet coaching 232–8
intimacy with client, establishing 69
irrational beliefs 137, 138, 157–9,
    162

journalling 92–4, 191

kinesthetic learners 74
Kolb's learning styles model 75

laser coaching 224–5
lateral approaches to clients 58
leap coaching 82
learned responses 62
learning, facilitating 71–3
learning styles models 73–6
letter-writing 93–4, 171
lifestyle changes 39–40
light 63
linear coaching 83
list-making 93
listening, active 69–70, 113–16
lists of resources 234
LOH (Likelihood of Hospitalization)
    prediction model 24–5

marketing plans
  anticipating market changes 255
  competitive analysis 254
  industry analysis 251–2
  market segments 252
  market trends and growth rates
    254
  marketing strategy 255
  target markets 252–4
marketing wellness coaching
  consumer buying behaviour
    239–43
  creating a marketing plan 251–5
  ideas for 244–51
  selling emotional concepts 243–4
mature learner study coaching 208
MBSR (mindfulness-based stress
    reduction) 193–4
meaning, finding 60
medical monitors 23
medical qigong 190–1
medical wellness 37
medication adherence study 25–6
meditation 151, 186–7, 211
membership sites 235–6
'Memo' 21

memory enhancement 23
men, coaching for 203–4, 208
mental health coaching 206
mentoring principles 67–8
metaphors, use of 130–1
MI (motivational interviewing) 81
mindbody integration
  mindbody solutions 54
  and PNI development 46–50
  and stress 50–4
mindfulness 60, 151, 193–4
mindsets
  client 54–63, 88–9, 90–1, 128
  conventional and complementary
    healthcare 32–3
mirroring technique 110, 118
MMT (multimodal therapy) 193
modelling 167
motivation 57, 84–9, 128, 240–1
motivational interviewing 81

nature and wellness coaching 208
NCCAM (National Center for
    Complementary and
    Alternative Medicine) 17–18,
    29
negotiated tasks 147, 176–7
networks 94–6
New Horizons programme 16
newsletters 218, 237
NHS (National Health Service)
    16–17
  and Bupa's Collaborative Care
    Model 25
  community health coaches 27
niche markets 197–9, 201–2
  creating a diverse business model
    213–20
  ideas for 202–13
  plan to find a niche 220–1
  products and services 200–1
  researching trends 199–200
NLP (neuro-linguistic programming)
    192
nurse robots 24
nutrition 185–6, 212–13

occupational wellness 39
online coaching 206, 219, 232–3

pain management 187–8
PAM (Patient Activation Measure)
    26–7
pancreas system, artificial 23
paradigm coaching 82
paradox coaching 83
paraphrasing 114
parenting coaching 212
partnership niche 202
patches 24
performance coaching 82
person-centred therapy 40–1
personal evolution 83
personal foundation model 82

personal responsibility questions
    111–12
Philips Heart Start Automatic
    External Defibrillator 20
Phillips iPill 24
philosophical pathways 59
physical wellness 37
pie charts 165
planning 72, 78, 152–3, 153, 154
  see also action planning
PMR (progressive muscle relaxation)
    182–3
PNI (psychoneuroimmunology)
    development 46–50
positive ageing see ageing
positive psychology 191–2
positivity 61
posture, as means of expression 110
powerful questioning 70, 111–13
practitioner therapy 40–1
precedents, identifying 201
pregnancy coaching 211–12
presence, establishing a coaching 69
preventative approach 43–4
print copies 236
private healthcare 18–19
procrastination 85–9
products and services
  effects of food industry on 14
  ideas for 202–13, 213–20
  improving 200–1
  sectors for 13
progress management 72–3, 177–8
psychological wellness 36
psychology
  humanistic 183–4
  positive 191–2
purchase options 242–3
PWP (Personal Wellness Plan)
    122–3, 125

qigong 190–1
quality of life coaching 83
questioning
  effective 146–7
  faulty thinking 159
  powerful 70, 111–13
  WHAT coaching model 80–1
questionnaire, learning styles 76

rapport building 58, 116–19
realistic, helping client to be 61
REBT (rational emotive behaviour
    therapy) 189
recovery coaching 83
referral 172–5
referrals 247
reflecting feelings 115
reflective writing 93
Reiki 187
rejection, fear of 87–8
relationships coaching 212
relationships, fear of 87
relaxation response 48, 50
relaxation techniques 167, 182–3

religious pathways 59
remote coaching 228–38
repeat business 238
reports 220, 235
resistance, overcoming 159–63
resource lists 234
response cost 167
response prevention 167
responsibility 33, 56, 111–12
retreats 210, 216–17
reviews 233
RIBA (Robot for Interactive Body Assistance) 24
role-play 165

sceptical clients 62–3
screening 214
self-comparisons 165, 172
self-disclosure 130
self-discovery 61
self-esteem 58, 130
self-monitoring and recording 167
self-nourishment 59
self-responsibility 56
services *see* products and services
sexuality 212
shadow 63
shift coaching 83
shopping trends 21–2
skills coaching 131–2
SMART goals 76–7, 123–4, 152
smoking cessation coaching 206
social networking 95–6
social skills coaching 166
social wellness 37–8
software 219
solution coaching 82
solution-focused brief therapy 189
spa treatments 20, 208, 216–17
Spain, Bupa in 25
specification questions 112
spiritual pathways 59
spiritual wellness 34–5, 208, 217
sports coaching 205–6
standards, professional 68
STEPPPA coaching model 79–80
stick-on patches 24
stimulus control 167
strategic alliances, building 249
strategic business networking 96
strategic coaching 82
stress
    acute and chronic 50–1

and change 51–2
    effects on health 52–4
    signs of *51*
stress management 181, 210–11
SUCCESS coaching model 78–9
success, fear of 87
support for clients 94
synergy 78

TA (transactional analysis) 189
TATT (Tired All The Time) Syndrome 22
tactile learners 74
talking to boss scenario 175
target markets 252–4
task delegation scenario 173–4
tasks, negotiated 147, 176–7
technology for wellness 22
tele-coaching 228–31
tele-seminars 230–1, 251
thinking, faulty
    irrational beliefs 137, *138*, 157–9, *162*
    overcoming client resistance 159–63
    reduction of distress 172–5
    tools for use with client 164–72
    see also mindsets: client
thoughts
    links between emotions and behaviours *144*
    stopping obsessive 171
time management 174–5, 211
tiredness 22
traditional coaching 83
training 215–16
training manuals 219
transactional analysis (TA) 189
transition 56
travel with wellness coach 210
trust of client, establishing 69
turnaround coaching 82
tutorials 219

uncertainty, managing 57
uncommitted clients 60

VARK model of learning 74, 118
vision coaching 83
visual learners 74
visualization 184–5
voice, as means of expression 109
vulnerability, expressing 61

web-based wellness centre 206
webcam coaching 232–3
weight management coaching 207
weighting 165
wellness
    consumer spending on 21–2
    defining 31–2
    eclectic approach to 30–1
    growth of the industry 11–15
    six areas of 33–40, *34*
    technology 22
wellness coaching
    agreements 68, *107*
    balance with counselling 41–2, 45, 128–9
    as business expansion idea 213
    competencies 68–73
    effect on DM outcomes 26–7
    eight-step process to using CBC in 139–43
    ending the coaching relationship 132
    facilitating opening session 121–4, *125–7*
    facilitating subsequent sessions 128–31
    ideas for 202–13, 213–20, 244–51
    integrated approach 40–5, 63–4, *64*
    integrating complementary therapies 46
    marketing 251–5
    models 76–84
    networks 94–6
    principles 66–7
    programmes 233
    short- or long-term 202
    Wellness Coaching Intro-Pack 101–2, *103–6*
WHAT coaching model 80–1
will 77
women, coaching for 203
work interruptions scenario 172–3
workouts 22
workshops 225–7
writing as therapy 93
    see also journalling

young people coaching 202–3

Zen coaching 82

Author Index

ABC Business Consulting 251
Abrams, M. 158
Adams, K. 93
Ader, R. 48, 49
American Institute of Stress 53
Association for Applied
    Psychophysiology and
    Biofeedback 180–1
Association of Humanistic
    Psychology Practitioners 183

BCC Research 22
Beard, G. 47
Beary, J.F. 48
Beck, A. 135, 145–6
Beck, J. 159, 160, 163
Benson, H. 48
Beutler, L.E. 160
Beveridge, W. 16
Birk, L. 48
British Association for Applied
    Nutrition and Nutritional
    Therapy 185
British Autogenic Society 182
British Society for Ecological
    Medicine 190
British Society of Integrated
    Medicine 30
Bruce, R. 93
Bupa 25

Cabot, R.C. 47
Cannon, W.B. 47
Carol, M.P. 48
CBC News 23
Cohen, N. 48, 49
Craig, G. 191
Csikszentmihalyi, M. 191–2

Downey, M. 77
Dryden, W. 141, 169, 170, 189
Dunn, L.H. 31, 48

eHealthNews 19
Ellis, A. 135, 137
Engel, G.L. 49

Faculty of Integrated Medicine 30
Felten, D.N. 49
Fenton, S. 15
Fleming, N.D. 74, 118
Furlong, M. 15

Goodman, P. 188
Gregorc, A.F. 73

Hales, D. 52
Hefferline, R. 188
Hettler, B. 34
Holmes, O.W. 44
Holmes, T.H. 51
Honey, P. 76
Hubel, D.H. 149

Imperial College Healthcare NHS
    Trust 12
Institute for Solution-Focused
    Therapy 189
Institute of Medicine 17
International Coach Federation 68
Izzard, J. 19

Jacobson, E. 47, 182, 189
Joines, V. 189

Kiecolt-Glaser, J.K. 52–3

Lindahl, K. 113
Luthe, W. 182

MarketsandMarkets 15
Maslow, A. 84, 183, 241
Mason, R.O. 91
Mathison, J. 192
Mayer, J. 188
McLeod, A. 79
Medical News Today 26
Medical Wellness Association 37
Melko, C. 26
Miller, C. 38
Miller, N.E. 48
Miller, W.J. 47
Miller, W.R. 81
Mills, C. 74
Mindful Living Programs 193
Moleiro, C. 160
Moos, R.H. 48
Mumford, A. 76

National Center for Complementary
    and Alternative Medicine
    (NCCAM) 17, 29, 186–7
Neenan, M. 141, 189
NHS West Essex 27

O'Donnell 32

Ornish, D. 37

Palmer, S. 24, 164, 169, 170, 193
Pelletier, K. 54
Perls, F. 188
Pert, C.B. 49
Pilates, J.H. 47
Pilzer, P.Z. 31
Progoff, I. 94

Rahe, R.H. 51
Ries, A. 200
Ries, L. 200
Rochester Review 49
Rogers, C. 40
Rowe, A.J. 91
Ruff, M. 49

Salovey, P. 188
Schultz, J.H. 182
Seligman, M.E.P 191–2
Selye, H. 47
Siegelman, E. 52
Snyderman, R. 29–30
Solomon, G.F. 48
Sperry, R.W. 149
Spiegel, D. 53
Stewart, I. 189
Stratmann, L. 25

Talebi, H. 160
The Cochrane Collaboration 17
The Hartman Group 21
Thomas, W. 79
Toffler, A. 51
Tosey, P. 192
Trend Hunter Magazine 20–1, 24
Tubbs, I. 24

United Nations 22

Vale, M. 27

Wasik, B. 139
Weil, A.T. 29–30
Wein, H. 53
What's Next 21, 22, 23
Whitmore, J. 76
Whybrow, A. 24
Wiesel, T.N. 149
Wolff, H.G. 47
Wolpe, J. 135
World Health Organization 31, 32